Research Methods and Audit in General Practice

SECOND EDITION

Oxford General Practice Series · 29

DAVID ARMSTRONG
Reader in Sociology as applied to Medicine
Department of General Practice
United Medical and Dental Schools of
Guy's and St Thomas's Hospitals

JOHN GRACE
General Practitioner
Higham, Kent

OXFORD   NEW YORK   TOKYO
OXFORD UNIVERSITY PRESS
1994

Oxford University Press, Walton Street, Oxford OX2 6DP
Oxford   New York
Athens   Auckland   Bangkok   Bombay
Calcutta   Cape Town   Dar es Salaam   Delhi
Florence   Hong Kong   Istanbul   Karachi
Kuala Lumpur   Madras   Madrid   Melbourne
Mexico City   Nairobi   Paris   Singapore
Taipei   Tokyo   Toronto
and associated companies in
Berlin   Ibadan

Oxford is a trade mark of Oxford University Press

Published in the United States
by Oxford University Press Inc., New York

A catalogue record for this book is available from the British Library

Library of Congress Cataloging in Publication Data
Armstrong, David, 1947 June 3–
Research methods and audit on general practice/David Armstrong.
(Oxford medical publications)   (Oxford general
practice series; no. 29)
Includes bibliographical references and index.
1. Medicine–Research–Methodology.   2. Medical audit.   I. Grace, John, MRCGP.
II. Title.   III. Series.   IV. Series: Oxford general practice series; no. 29
R850.A75   1994   610'.72–dc20   94–21988
ISBN 0 19 262454 7

Typeset by Advance Typesetting Ltd, Oxon
Printed in Great Britain by
Redwood Books, Trowbridge, Wilts

Preface

The aim of this book is to provide sufficient practical guidance to get you to the point where you will be able to complete and publish a research project of your own. We have therefore tried to emphasize involvement in actually doing research: in part this is through examples and also by various assignments:

1. At various points in the text you will find *Questions*: you may like to pause here and see if you can answer them. The text then goes on to provide answers which you can compare with your own.

2. At other points you will find *Exercises*: these are meant to be an assessment of what you have learned. In the first read-through you may wish to skip them but later you may wish to try and complete them.

3. We have also included some suggested *Tasks* at the end of every chapter, that you can carry out on your own, or preferably with others. In fact, as research is so often a group activity you might consider working through this book with others, perhaps carrying out a 'group research project' as you do so, that way you would be able to share the discussion and the work. Perhaps a trainers' workshop, a young principals' group, or a trainer and trainee might find working together on a research question of mutual interest a useful way of both learning about and doing research.

The research process

The different stages of carrying out a research project will be covered in the various chapters of this book. In outline these stages are:

- asking a question
- establishing a plan or design of how the answering is to proceed. This is the guide for all future activity
- deciding how the various ideas expressed in the question are to be measured
- doing the measuring—usually referred to as 'data collection'
- organizing the collected data into a form suitable for analysis
- analysing the data, usually with the involvement of statistical tests and a computer
- writing up the results
- if appropriate, finding a journal in which to publish the study.

The penultimate chapter, on writing a research protocol, could equally well have been the first chapter because the protocol comes near the start of all research projects. In the end we thought that knowing how to begin should probably come after seeing where you were going to go: writing a protocol is therefore at the end, but we hope that it is the beginning of your research in the rich and varied field of general practice.

For this second edition we have revised the text and added two new chapters. One, on using the Epi Info data analysis package, recognizes that computers are so often used today in data analysis and this particular package is a useful—and free—facility for exploring general practice data. The second additional chapter, on carrying out audit in general practice, is an acknowledgement of the import-ance of this activity in general practice. Many audit skills are also research skills, so this concluding chapter attempts to place the preceding chapters in an audit context, pointing out the similarities as well as differences in the two processes.

We have valued the suggestions of a number of GPs who commented to us on the first edition. Also, we would particularly like to thank our colleague, Professor Michael Calnan, who was a co-author of the earlier edition of this text: despite the revision his important contribution to the original still informs much of what follows.

London   D.A.
June 1994   J.G.

Contents

1 Asking questions

This first chapter is about the most fundamental part of 'doing' research, namely asking questions. Research attempts to answer questions: this is both very simple and very important. Possibly one of the commonest reasons for research 'failing' is that the project did not start with a proper question. Deciding to 'look at' an area or problem, or collecting data about something that seems interesting, is, by and large, wasted time. *Research must start with a question.* This point cannot be reiterated sufficiently; do not start 'doing' research until you have a question.

The difficulty with this part of the research process is that it cannot be taught in the conventional sense. In many ways this is the personal and creative component of research that comes from you. However, this first chapter will provide some suggestions of how to start the question-asking process and offer basic guidelines to enable you to decide whether the question you ask is a good one or not.

THINKING OF QUESTIONS

Research is often described as concerned with testing theories or hypotheses. A hypothesis (or theory) is a statement of sets of ideas or concepts. Thus: 'Patients without appointments are more likely to present psychosocial problems' is a hypothesis about the world that research might be expected to show as either true or false. (Note that any research hypothesis can just as easily, and perhaps more helpfully, be expressed as a research question: 'Are patients without appointments more likely to present psychosocial problems?') The hypothesis or question is then tested in the 'real' world of facts and data (perhaps a questionnaire to patients both with and without appointments, and then compare the two groups). Hence science has been characterized as the 'hypothetico-deductive method' because an event is deduced from an abstract hypothesis and the real world examined to see if it is there or has occurred: if it has, the hypothesis is said to have been confirmed. The hypothesis or question is thus the starting point for research and, as has been stressed, is therefore very important. Nevertheless it is only the *formal* starting point.

In popular imagery the scientist always starts from the question or the theory that happens to come as a flash of inspiration, usually in the bath or on a tram (when they were around). The reality is far less romantic. Most research questions actually arise from rather routine observed events. Doll and Hill did not suddenly think 'Does smoking cause lung cancer?'. Clinicians had already observed an apparent link between the behaviour and the disease in the patients they treated. This was induction: observations leading to a question. Thereafter the question was treated by the canons of scientific procedure, namely the hypothetico-deductive method, in that a study was set up to compare the smoking habits of patients with and without lung cancer. Science moves in a continuous process of induction from experience followed by formal deduction and testing, followed by further induction, and so on.

In recent years the emphasis on deduction as the key formal method of science has been challenged. There is now increasing acceptance for formalizing the inductive process as a proper scientific activity: thus the generation of research questions can be also be viewed as a scientific process. This latter approach to research is encompassed within so-called qualitative research methods that attempt to work from the data to the hypothesis rather than the other way round. Both traditional quantitative methods and the newer qualitative ones are covered in this book, though the emphasis is on the former.

In terms of the constant movement from induction to deduction and back again, the practical message is that by and large research questions do not come from some nebulous faculty either possessed or not possessed, such as creativity or inspiration, but from everyday observations. In formulating questions anything goes: use clinical experience, chance findings, casual discussions, car rides, and toy boat in the bath, but get the questions flowing. Keep a book, a diary, a list: sort them, reject some, develop others, and when you have one which you find interesting consider putting it to the test.

Of course, having selected an interesting question one is still faced with the problem of whether the ability to answer that question is within the resources of time, money, support, and so on, available to you. A 'good' research question may not be synonymous with 'a good research question for a GP' or even 'a good research question for me'.

Another important point to make is that the questions need not necessarily be complicated or difficult. It is often the simple questions that are easily overlooked, or the answers assumed:

- are coronaries best managed in hospital?
- is shingles contagious?
- does physiotherapy help in the management of acute low back pain?

You do not have to be a creative genius to think of research questions. Suffice it to say that in the largely uncharted field of primary care a large number of questions or areas of doubt probably arise during the course of every working day to make the preparation of a list of questions relatively easy. That is not to say that what may appear to be easy questions to ask are necessarily easy questions to answer, but they may be. This book can help you to sift your ideas so as to eliminate obviously doubtful ones, and it can possibly help you work out what to do next. But it is your ability to recognize areas of doubt and turn them into good questions that will ultimately determine whether you do 'good' research no matter how many 'techniques' you master. The questions are there: just open your mind and let the questions creep in!

EXERCISE 1.1

You may find it worthwhile to take a notebook with you on your next full working day. During the course of the day jot down in the book ten questions or areas of doubt that occur to you. At the end of the day subject these questions to a critical analysis to separate out those questions that might be suitable for researching further. Evaluate them in terms of answerability and general usefulness. You could use a scale of 1 to 5 for each characteristic, marking the least answerable and the least useful as 1, the most answerable and the most useful as 5, and using 2, 3, and 4 for points in between.

Questions	Answerability	Usefulness

QUESTION 1.1

Which of the following questions, the sort that might occur to you during the course of a day's work, might be suitable as the basis for a research project?

- Does smoking cause cancer?
- Did Mr Smith take his tablets today?
- Is this pain angina?
- I wonder if God helps recovery from surgery?
- Are antibiotics effective against viruses?
- Does bed rest help in the treatment of bad backs?
- Do chronic bronchitics cough up sputum?

- *Does smoking cause cancer?* It is already well established and proven beyond all reasonable doubt that there is a strong association between smoking and several types of cancer. A compromise has to be reached between attempts to re-invent the wheel and a proper questioning of established but unproven practices. In this particular instance the balance would appear to be clearly on the side of the wheelsmith.
- *Did Mr Smith take his tablets today?* Some questions, although possibly of interest in a particular instance, are of limited general applicability and can be considered too trivial for the use of the research method as a way of answering them.
- *Is this pain angina?* This is the type of question that occurs in everyday clinical practice. However, it requires the application of the clinical, rather than the research, method. Whilst, as will be discussed later, there are strong similarities

in approach between the two methods, the research method is best reserved for questions that appear to have a wider application.

• *I wonder if God helps recovery from surgery?* This is obviously an important question. It is also of wide application. Unfortunately it is unanswerable as it stands. If it were rephrased as 'Does a belief in God aid recovery from surgery?' then the question is limited to one of more manageable proportions, although it would then be a matter of judgement as to whether the amended question is now so altered as to have little in common with the original proposal. To reiterate, at the end of the day a good research question has to be answerable.

• *Are antibiotics effective against viruses?* This really is a similar problem to the question about smoking and cancer. The answer is already known beyond reasonable doubt. However your observations may lead you to question the assumed answer and formulate new hypotheses—but are you sure there is not an alternative simple explanation?

• *Does bed rest help in the treatment of bad backs?* This is a question of wide general application which tests an accepted clinical practice for which there does not appear to be a lot of evidence. This could well form the basis for a useful research question.

• *Do chronic bronchitics cough up sputum?* This is essentially a definitional question. The accepted definition of chronic bronchitis is based on the regular expectoration of a defined amount of sputum. Therefore there is no real question to answer.

In summary, questions can be rendered inappropriate for research because:

• The answer is already known
• The question is not of general interest, possibly only related to one case
• Some questions, although important, are unanswerable by research methods used and accepted at present
• Some questions are definitional.

Let us examine this last point in more detail.

EMPIRICAL QUESTIONS

Questions and answers can be divided into two sorts: *definitional* ones that simply restate in other words the initial idea, and *empirical* ones that potentially tell something about the world in which we live. Karl Popper, the doyen of scientific philosophers, used this idea in his criterion of what was to count as a scientific statement or question. He decided that science consists of questions, hypotheses, and statements that are, *in principle*, refutable, that is contain the potential of being disproved.

Be careful therefore to distinguish between these two claims to the truth. This book is only concerned with empirical questions and not those that are definitional—though sometimes the latter can masquerade as the former.

For example, could you investigate the claim that 'asthma causes recurrent small airways obstruction' or that 'asthma stunts growth'? Probably not the former, since if asthma did not cause recurrent small airways obstruction then it would not, by definition, be asthma; but the second hypothesis can be investigated because it could be incorrect *without* undermining the accepted definition of asthma.

Sometimes it is unclear whether a question is 'true by definition' or empirically testable. Consider the following questions:

- Do patients with over 95 mm Hg diastolic blood pressure have hypertension?
- Are patients who appear reluctant to return to work malingerers?
- Are diabetics with a fasting blood sugar of 8 mmol/litre adequately controlled?

In each case the question might be a definitional one, that is if hypertension, malingering, and diabetic control are pre-defined. On the other hand, if these three phenomena are defined in some other independent way it may be possible to 'test' the question. For example, if hypertension were defined as raised blood pressure such as to increase the risk of a stroke then it would be possible to test whether 95 mm Hg diastolic pressure was an indicator of hypertension.

EXERCISE 1.2

Which of the following questions would be suitable for a research project?

1. Do diabetics have high fasting blood sugars?
2. Do NSAIs (non-steroidal anti-inflammatory agents) cause cancer?
3. Are patients who complain of dizziness likely to suffer from a serious disease?
4. Are my receptionists kind to my patients?
5. Am I working harder than my partners?
6. Is asthma more common in only children?

Suggested answers are found at the end of the chapter.

A NOTE ON AUDIT

The activity of audit is very closely related to research, and indeed, often gets confused with it. Audit is usually taken to mean a measurement of performance against a predetermined set of standards. For example one could decide that for a diagnosis of hypertension to be confirmed, three readings of a diastolic pressure over 100 mm Hg on three separate occasions were required. An auditing exercise of all the patients on anti-hypertensive treatment could be carried out, in order to determine to what extent this pre-set standard for the diagnosis had been satisfied. Therefore, in doing an audit there are opportunities for using many research skills, particularly in devising standards and monitoring performance. However, the audit process is targeted at a different goal to that of research. The latter is concerned with improving understanding of the world, whether through testing hypotheses or generating interesting descriptions (through qualitative methods), while the former is concerned with introducing change into a little corner of that world. Audit is carried out with the express purpose of changing things if they do not measure up to the agreed standard; research may have implications for change, but does not of itself say how the world should be.

The process of carrying out an audit is described in Chapter 12, but many of the research skills outlined in the intervening chapters will facilitate audit activity.

EXERCISE 1.3

Which of the following questions belong to research and which to audit?

1. Is my prescribing rate higher than that of other GPs in my area?
2. Does recent unemployment make patients attend more often?
3. Is my appointment system operating satisfactorily?
4. Do people who have to look after dependent relations at home consult more often?
5. Are the immunization rates for my 5-year-olds satisfying the district norms?

Suggested answers are to be found at the end of the chapter.

EXPLORING THE QUESTION

Having identified a possibly 'good' research question, the next stage is to investigate the background of the question. Has someone else had a go at answering it? Is the answer known? Has someone formulated it in a better way?

In addition, this exploratory phase will be useful for the very final stages of the research process, namely in writing up for publication, in that a journal article usually opens with some discussion of the background to the question together with an overview of existing literature (see Chapter 10).

Let us examine the background to a simple question.

QUESTION 1.2

Are antibiotics of value in the treatment of acute otitis media?

• yes
• no
• sometimes.

Consider the grounds you have for holding your opinion, the degree of certainty with which you hold it, and possible sources of knowledge. How could you find out whether an adequate answer already exists for this or any other particular problem? There are many fairly readily available sources of knowledge that are commonly used depending on the question being asked and the degree of faith in the received answer.

1. *Ask a GP colleague*? This is easy, and possibly the most widely used method; but how reliable is it? Is the opinion of a colleague likely to be based on similar false assumptions to your own?

2. *Look it up in a textbook*? Textbooks are extremely useful and again fairly readily available sources of information. They vary greatly in standard and size, depending partly on the audience for which they were designed. A 100-page *Concise illustrated textbook of ear, nose, and throat medicine for students and GPs* has to sacrifice for the sake of brevity certain aspects of erudition that a 1000-page *Textbook on disease of the human cochlear* does not. Shorter tomes are more likely to be a synopsis of common practice rather than valid statements of current knowledge. They are rarely referenced, so making it difficult if not impossible for the reader to check the information presented. All textbooks also suffer from preparation-lag; the often considerable delay between the writing and the publishing means that the information can be anything up to two years out of date on the day the brand new textbook is published.

3. *Ask a consultant colleague in the field*? This is likely to produce a more authoritative opinion or answer than asking a non-specialist colleague. It should also be based on more recent developments or information than textbooks—on the assumption that specialists read specialists' journals. But can you be any more certain that it is more reliable? If the opinion is backed by references that can be checked, then one might perhaps be less suspicious, but unfortunately people develop ways of behaving and doing things that they find comfortable. Doctors are no exception. Many become entrapped in a mode of unquestioning behaviour where doubt does not assume a prominent place. Comments about the level of research activity in primary care, and among GPs in particular, could probably as readily be made about in-post consultants outside academic units. Indeed very few aspects of clinical practice have ever been subjected to proper scientific evaluation. With these reservations in mind it may be that specialists are a source of information that needs to be subjected to as much critical assessment as any other.

4. *Carry out a literature review*? To find the current state of play about most medical problems one is forced to 'search the literature'—that is, either to find a detailed critical review article on a subject with references appended, or to look up the original article itself and to make some evaluative assessment of that article, especially in relation to the specific problem you have in mind. This usually entails spending time in your local postgraduate centre library. These of course vary greatly in size and facilities. A possible minimal criterion of the adequacy of your local postgraduate centre library would be whether or not it has a qualified librarian. If it has not, then you might benefit from finding the nearest

one that has. Librarians are highly trained specialists in finding things out, and a few minutes discussing the problem you are trying to solve with a librarian may well increase the efficiency of the time you actually spend searching in the library many times over. Get to know your library and the facilities it offers: it is a valuable resource.

The librarian will probably introduce you to two methods of searching through the literature.

(a) *Manual literature searches.* These are normally carried out by looking up the topic in *Cumulated Index Medicus.* This is an index, or list, of all papers published in the major medical journals throughout the world. It appears monthly, with yearly compilations, catalogued by both subject and author. The use of *Index Medicus* involves:

• finding the right synonym for the key word or words, under which heading papers relating to your particular query might be filed
• looking at this key word in the Subject Headings.

It is especially worth looking for review articles in the leading and readily available journals (such as the *British Medical Journal, British Journal of General Practice, Lancet,* for example). Once into these articles a form of journal daisy chaining can be started. The particular article is looked up in the named journal, and then further papers listed in the references at the end of the article can be examined. One or two might be obtained and the reference lists of these in turn can be looked at, the papers examined and so on, and so on ....

Obviously papers in the English language, and especially British journals, will be easier to obtain, but the librarian should be able to obtain a copy of most papers on request.

For example, to answer the question of whether antibiotics are of value in the treatment of otitis media requires the following procedure:

Look up the keyword 'Otitis Media'. In this example, this was done using the *Cumulated Index Medicus* for 1985. In a sub-division of the entries under 'Otitis Media', sub-titled 'Drug Therapy', were found six articles that seemed to address the question posed. Two of these, an original article and a letter criticizing the article, were in the *British Medical Journal,* commonly available in most medical libraries. The references at the bottom of this article produced further articles, and further references lists and so on.

Figures 1.1 and 1.2 illustrate this procedure.

(b) *Computerized literature searches.* This is the age of the technological and information revolution. As well as blasting aliens, the computer in its spare time is used for the storage of vast amounts of information and, more importantly, allows ready access to and searching of this information. This facility has been seized upon by those engaged in compiling catalogues such as the Index Medicus.

1985 **CUMULATED INDEX MEDICUS** **OTITIS MEDIA**

PG. **Mykosen** 1985 May;28(5):234–7

Bacteriologic studies in external otitis in Dar es Salaam, Tanzania. Manni JJ, et al. **Trop Geogr Med** 1984 Sep; 36(3):293–5

PARASITOLOGY

[Human otoacariasis caused by Otobius megnini in Calama, Chile] Burchard L, et al. **Bol Chil Parasitol** 1984 Jan-Jun; 39(1-2):15–6 (Eng. Abstr.) **(Spa)**

PATHOLOGY

Bilateral chondrodermatitis helicis: case presentation and literature review. Cannon CR. **Am J Otol** 1985 Mar; 6(2):164–6

RADIOGRAPHY

Radiologic abnormalities of malignant otitis externa. Pripstein S, et al. **Rev Laryngol Otol Rhinol (Bord)** 1984; 105(3):307-10

Radiologic evaluation of malignant external otitis. Smoker WR, et al. **Rev Laryngol Otol Rhinol (Bord)** 1984; 105(3):297-301

RADIONUCLIDE IMAGING

The radionuclide diagnosis, evaluation and follow-up of malignant external otitis (MEO). The value of immediate blood pool scanning. Garty I, et al. **J Laryngol Otol** 1985 Feb;99(2):109-15

RADIOTHERAPY

[Low-energy laser irradiation in the complex treatment of patients with ear diseases] Bykov VL, et al. **Vopr Kurortol Fizioter Lech Fiz Kult** 1985 Mar-Apr; (2):60–2 **(Rus)**

THERAPY

Prognostic implications of therapy for necrotizing external otitis [clinical conference] Corey JP, et al. **Am J Otol** 1985 Jul;6(4):353-8

Surgical applications of the expandable ear wick. Cannon CR. **Laryngoscope** 1985 Jun;95(6):739–40

VETERINARY

Mycotic otitis externa in animals. Kuttin ES, et al. **Mykosen** 1985 Feb;28(2):61-8

OTITIS MEDIA

Experimental otitis media with effusion. Proceedings of the international conference, Lövångers Kyrkstad, August 17-20, 1983. **Acta Otolaryngol [Suppl] (Stockh)** 1984; 414:1-188

Recent advances in otitis media with effusion. Report of research conference. Fort Lauderdale, May 20-21, 1983. **Ann Otol Rhinol Laryngol [Suppl]** 1985 Jan-Feb;116:1-32

A 5-year prospective case-control study of the influence of early otitis media with effusion on reading achievement. Lous J, et al. **Int J Pediatr Otorhinolaryngol** 1984 Oct; 8(1):19-30

Persistent and recurrent otitis media. A review of the 'otitis-prone' condition. Berman S, et al. **Primary Care** 1984 Sep;11(3):407-17 (57 ref.)

[Serous-mucoid otitis media in infants] Narcy P, et al. **Ann Pediatr (Paris)** 1984 Dec;31(11):939-43 (Eng. Abstr.) **(Fre)**

[Otitis media in the newborn infant: cytologic and bacteriologic study and long-term results] Pestalozza G, et al. **Acta Otorhinolaryngol Ital** 1984 Jan-Feb;4(1):27–47 (Eng. Abstr.) **(Ita)**

BLOOD

Subclinical trace element deficiency in children with undue susceptibility to infections. Bondestam M, et al. **Acta Paediatr Scand** 1985 Jul;74(4):515-20

Similar hematologic changes in children receiving trimethoprim-sulfamethoxazole or amoxicillin for otitis media. Feldman S, et al. **J Pediatr** 1985 Jun;106(6):995-1000

CHEMICALLY INDUCED

[Carrageenins-induced otitis media in animal] Shibahara Y, et al. **Nippon Jibiinkoka Gakkai Kaiho** 1984 Jun;87(6):680–7 (Eng. Abstr.) **(Jpn)**

COMPLICATIONS

Middle ear disease in samples from the general population. II. History of otitis and otorrhea in relation to tympanic membrane pathology. The study of men born in 1913 and 1923. Rudin R, et al. **Acta Otolaryngol (Stockh)** 1985 Jan-Feb;99(1-2):53-9

Intracranial complications of otitis media. Debruyne F. **Acta Otorhinolaryngol Belg** 1984;38(2):128-32

Characteristics of earache among children with acute otitis media. Hayden GF, et al. **Am J Dis Child** 1985 Jul; 139(7):721-3

The frequency of vestibular disorders in developmentally delayed preschoolers with otitis media. Schaaf RC. **Am J Occup Ther** 1985 Apr;39(4):247-52

Subarachnoid space: middle ear pathways and recurrent meningitis. Barcz DV, et al. **Am J Otol** 1985 Mar; 6(2):157–63

The etiologic role of acute suppurative otitis media in chronic secretory otitis. Stangerup SE, et al. **Am J Otol** 1985 Mar; 6(2):126–31

Sensorineural hearing loss in otitis media. Paparella MM, et al. **Ann Otol Rhinol Laryngol** 1984 Nov-Dec;93(6 Pt 1):623-9

Ventilating tubes in the middle ear. Long-term observations. Gundersen T, et al. **Arch Otolaryngol** 1984 Dec; 110(12):783–4

Analysis of fifty cases of facial palsy due to otitis media. Takahashi H, et al. **Arch Otorhinolaryngol** 1985; 241(2):163-8

Otitis media: the role of speech-language pathologists. Garrard KR, et al. **ASHA** 1985 Jul;27(7):35-9

The minimally hearing-impaired child. Bess FH. **Ear Hear** 1985 Jan-Feb;6(1):43-7

Basal cell carcinoma following chronic otitis media. Myskowski PL, et al. **Int J Dermatol** 1985 Mar;24(2):120–1

Brain abscess secondary to otitis media. Bradley PJ, et al. **J Laryngol Otol** 1984 Dec;98(12):1185-91

Lateral sinus thrombosis in the eighties. Debruyne F. **J Laryngol Otol** 1985 Jan;99(1):91-3

Otologic features of bacterial meningitis of childhood. Eavey RD, et al. **J Pediatr** 1985 Mar;106(3):402-7

Relationship between acute suppurative otitis media and chronic secretory otitis media: role of antibiotics. Mills R, et al. **J R Soc Med** 1984 Sep;77(9):754-7

Otitic hydrocephalus. Lenz RP, et al. **Laryngoscope** 1984 Nov;94(11 Pt 1):1451–4

Acute mastoiditis complicated by bacterial meningitis. Braverman AC, et al. **Mo Med** 1985 Jun;82(6):308-11

Purulent otitis media--a 'silent' source of sepsis in the pediatric intensive care unit. Persico M, et al. **Otolaryngol Head Neck Surg** 1985 Jun;93(3):330–4

Postinflammatory ossicular fixation: CT analysis with surgical correlation. Swartz JD, et al. **Radiology** 1985 Mar; 154(3):697-700

Intracranial complications of ear disease in a pediatric population with special emphasis on subdural effusion and empyema. Gower DJ, et al. **South Med J** 1985 Apr; 78(4):429-34

[Results of tympanometry in infantile allergic rhinopathy] Corrias A, et al. **Minerva Pediatr** 1984 Nov 30; 36(22):1115-8 (Eng. Abstr.) **(Ita)**

[Otogenic intracranial complications--an ever-present problem] Janczewski G, et al. **Otolaryngol Pol** 1985; 39(1):7-18 (Eng. Abstr.) **(Pol)**

[Chronic purulent otitis media complicated by an extensive phlegmon of the neck] Bystrenin AV. **Vestn Otorinolaringol** 1985 May-Jun;(3):79-80 **(Rus)**

[Roentgenological diagnosis of labyrinthine fistulas in chronic suppurative otitis media] Kossovoi AL. **Vestn Otorinolaringol** 1985 Jan-Feb;(1):17-20 (Eng. Abstr.) **(Rus)**

[Social rehabilitation of patients in the late period after surgery for an otogenic brain abscess] Markin SA, et al. **Vestn Otorinolaringol** 1985 May-Jun;(3):36-9 (Eng. Abstr.) **(Rus)**

[Otogenic brain abscess in a child] Sal'nikova EA, et al. **Vestn Otorinolaringol** 1985 Mar-Apr;(2):58-60 **(Rus)**

[Cerebrovascular disorders and ischemic stroke in patients with chronic suppurative otitis media, simulating otogenic intracranial complications] Shuster MA, et al. **Vestn Otorinolaringol** 1985 Jan-Feb;(1):41–4 (Eng. Abstr.) **(Rus)**

DIAGNOSIS

Otitis media in early infancy. Papadeas VA, et al. **Am J Emerg Med** 1984 May;2(3):251-3

Aboriginal child health. Stuart J. **Aust Fam Physician** 1985 Jul;14(7):677-80

Follow-up visit after acute otitis media. Puczynski MS, et al. **Br J Clin Pract** 1985 Apr;39(4):132-4, 153

Ear wax and otitis media in children. Fairey A, et al. **Br Med J [Clin Res]** 1985 Aug 10;291(6492):387-8

Study of middle ear disease using tympanometry in general practice. Reves R, et al. **Br Med J [Clin Res]** 1985 Jun 29;290(6486):1953-6

Age-specific patterns of diagnosis of acute otitis media. McFadden DM, et al. **Clin Pediatr (Phila)** 1985 Oct; 24(10):571-5

Otitis media in newborn infants. Pestalozza G. **Int J Pediatr Otorhinolaryngol** 1984 Dec;8(2):109-24

Acoustic impedance measurement as screening procedure in children: discussion paper. Brooks DN. **J R Soc Med** 1985 Feb;78(2):119-21

Screening for middle ear fluid in an urban pre-school population. Paulman PM, et al. **Nebr Med J** 1984 Sep; 69(9):307

Acoustic reflectometry in the detection of middle ear effusion. Lampe RM, et al. **Pediatrics** 1985 Jul;76(1):75-8

[Acute inflammation of the middle ear] Feenstra L. **Ned Tijdschr Geneeskd** 1985 Mar 23;129(12):532-6 **(Dut)**

[Tympanometry under nitrous oxide anesthesia in cases of seromucous otitis] Coeckelenbergh A, et al. **Acta Otorhinolaryngol Belg** 1984;38(5):485-8 (Eng. Abstr.) **(Fre)**

[Embryonal rhabdomyosarcoma of the middle ear and mastoid simulating chronic otitis media] Shohet I, et al. **Harefuah** 1984 Nov 15;107(10):290–1 (Eng. Abstr.) **(Heb)**

[A case of aspergillosis of the ear] Sekula J, et al. **Otolaryngol Pol** 1985;39(2):166–70 (Eng. Abstr.) **(Pol)**

[Differential diagnostic problems in diseases and injuries of the middle ear] Kitanoski B, et al. **Vojnosanit Pregl** 1985 Jan-Feb;42(1):14–8 (Eng. Abstr.) **(Scr)**

DRUG THERAPY

Efficacy of Metronidazole in experimental Bacteroides fragilis otitis media. Thore M, et al. **Acta Otolaryngol (Stockh)** 1985 Jan-Feb;99(1-2):60–6

Acute otitis media in older children and adults treated with penicillin or erythromycin. Rosén C, et al. **Acta Otolaryngol [Suppl] (Stockh)** 1984;407:23-5

Antibiotic treatment of secretory otitis media. Sundberg L. **Acta Otolaryngol [Suppl] (Stockh)** 1984;407:26–9

Improving compliance with antibiotic regimens for otitis media. Randomized clinical trial in a pediatric clinic. Finney JW, et al. **Am J Dis Child** 1985 Jan;139(1):89-95

Erythromycin-sulfisoxazole vs amoxicillin in the treatment of acute otitis media in children. A double-blind, multiple-dose comparative study. Rodriguez WJ, et al. **Am J Dis Child** 1985 Aug;139(8):766–70

Drugs affecting clearance of middle ear secretions: a perspective for the management of otitis media with effusion. Brown DT, et al. **Ann Otol Rhinol Laryngol [Suppl]** 1985 Mar-Apr;117:3-15

Acute otitis media: a new treatment strategy [letter] **Br Med J [Clin Res]** 1985 Jun 8;290(6483):1743–4

Acute otitis media: a new treatment strategy. van Buchem FL, et al. **Br Med J [Clin Res]** 1985 Apr 6;290(6474):1033–7

The 'new' ampicillins: who needs them? Committee on Infectious Diseases and Immunization, Canadian Paediatric Society. **Can Med Assoc J** 1984 Nov 15;131(10):1223–4

Bromhexine in the treatment of otitis media with effusion. Stewart IA, et al. **Clin Otolaryngol** 1985 Jun;10(3):145-9

The long-term outcome of nonsuppurative otitis media with effusion. Dusdieker LB, et al. **Clin Pediatr (Phila)** 1985 Apr; 24(4):181-6

Fungal infection of the ear. Etiology and therapy with bifonazole cream or solution. Falser N. **Dermatologica** 1984; 169 Suppl 1:135–40

Oral nystatin [letter] Crook WG. **Ear Nose Throat J** 1985 Mar;64(3):155

Otitis media: treatment and side effects [letter] Crook WG. **Hosp Pract [Off]** 1985 Sep 30;20(9A):14, 16

Antimicrobial therapy of chronic otitis media with effusion. Healy GB. **Int J Pediatr Otorhinolaryngol** 1984 Oct; 8(1):13-7

Compliance with acute otitis media treatment. Reed BD, et al. **J Fam Pract** 1984 Nov;19(5):627-32

A randomized controlled trial of cefaclor compared with trimethoprim-sulfamethoxazole for treatment of acute otitis media. Marchant CD, et al. **J Pediatr** 1984 Oct;105(4):633-8

Mucolytic agents for glue ear [letter] Pearson JP, et al. **Lancet** 1985 Sep 21;2(8456):674

Trimet v amoxycillin in the treatment of otitis media in children [letter] Godfrey AA, et al. **NZ Med J** 1985 Apr 10;98(776):252

Medical management of serous otitis media. Crysdale WS. **Otolaryngol Clin North Am** 1984 Nov;17(4):653-7

Medical management of chronic otitis media. Jahn AF, et al. **Otolaryngol Clin North Am** 1984 Nov;17(4):673-7

Occurrence of Clostridium difficile toxin-associated gastroenteritis following antibiotic therapy for otitis media in young children. Hyams JS, et al. **Pediatr Infect Dis** 1984 Sep–Oct;3(5):433-6

In vivo sensitivity test in otitis media: efficacy of antibiotics. Howie VM, et al. **Pediatrics** 1985 Jan;75(1):8-13

Oral dexamethasone for treatment of persistent middle ear effusion. Macknin ML, et al. **Pediatrics** 1985 Feb; 75(2):329-35

Comparative treatment trial of augmentin versus cefaclor for acute otitis media with effusion. Odio CM, et al. **Pediatrics** 1985 May;75(5):819-26

Trimethoprim and amoxycillin in acute otitis media. Backhouse CI, et al. **Practitioner** 1985 Jan;229(1399):51–4

[Adapting the therapy to the course of acute otitis media] van Buchem FL, et al. **Ned Tijdschr Geneeskd** 1985 Jun 8;129(23):1093-9 (Eng. Abstr.) **(Dut)**

[Effect of Tavegyl (Polfa) on microorganisms detected in otocenosis during in vivo studies] Kurnatowski P, et al. **Otolaryngol Pol** 1984;38(3):219-24 (Eng. Abstr.) **(Pol)**

[Use of lekozim in middle ear diseases] Tarasov DI, et al. **Vestn Otorinolaringol** 1985 May-Jun;(3):43-7 (Eng. Abstr.) **(Rus)**

ENZYMOLOGY

Biochemical pathology of otitis media with effusion. Juhn SK, et al. **Acta Otolaryngol [Suppl] (Stockh)** 1984;414:45-51

Hydrolase activity in acute otitis media with effusion. Diven WF, et al. **Ann Otol Rhinol Laryngol** 1985 Jul-Aug;94(4 Pt 1):415-8

Antifibrinolytic activity in middle ear effusion. Hamaguchi Y, et al. **ORL J Otorhinolaryngol Relat Spec** 1984; 46(5):235-41

[Lysosomal enzyme activity in middle ear effusions] Hara A, et al. **Nippon Jibiinkoka Gakkai Kaiho** 1984 May; 87(5):596–602 (Eng. Abstr.) **(Jpn)**

ETIOLOGY

Endotoxin in middle ear effusions tested with Limulus assay.

12621

Fig. 1.1 Finding the references.

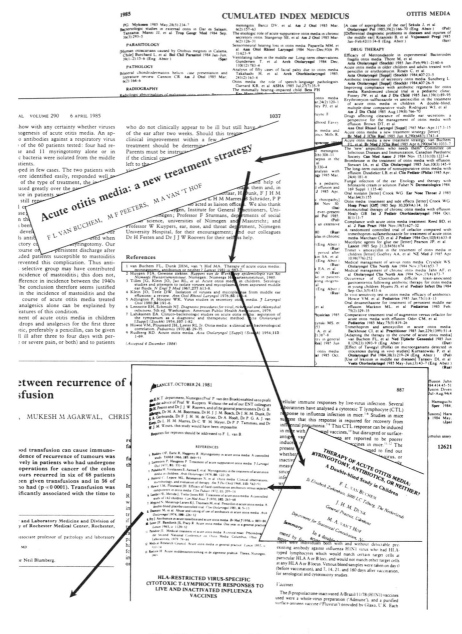

Fig. 1.2 Reference daisy-chaining.

There are several computerized databases solely restricted to medical literature. Many postgraduate centre libraries have facilities to plug into one of these centralized lists by using a computer terminal in the library and a telephone line connecting it to a large computer, often many thousands of miles away. The Royal College of General Practitioners provides a similar facility to both members and non-members (at different rates) with their ON-LINE SEARCH SERVICE. All these services provide a rapid search of a wide range of literature. They do have problems, however:

- They often cost money to use.
- The efficient use of the facility requires the correct selection of 'key words'. These are similar to those required for the manual use of *Index Medicus*, but need if anything to be even more specific and exact. For example using the key words 'ENT' and 'General Practice' to search the literature in the otitis media problem would provide a list of references of every publication on file, for as far back as has been computerized, in which any aspect of ENT was connected with any aspect of general practice.

The selection of the correct keywords is therefore the secret of using these databases. Again the librarian can be of enormous value in the proper selection of these keywords and the saving of your time and expense.

The medical librarian at a postgraduate centre was asked to produce a list of references that might help answer the question posed. The search was carried out on *Medline*, one of several computerized databases, using the keywords *otitis media* and *antibiotics*. The search was restricted to English-language journals for the past 5 years. It produced 52 articles.

QUESTION 1.3

What might be the respective advantages and disadvantages of manual and computerized literature searches?

The manual method might be expected to be time consuming and prone to errors. However, it allows discrimination in ignoring articles that address questions other than those in which one is directly interested, for example:

- Is drug A better than drug B in otitis media?
- Is 10 days of drug C better than 3 days?

It also allows one to ignore journals that are not immediately accessible. In the exercise described above, it was possible to identify two papers within 10 minutes, by van Buchem in the *British Medical Journal* and the *Lancet*, that appeared directly to address the question posed. The computerized search might be expected to be quicker and more thorough. In fact it took over a week to get the list back because of pressure of work on the librarian. It would have cost perhaps £20 and produced a far more comprehensive list, but in the end probably only 9 of the 52 papers were specifically looking at the question in hand; and for some reason it missed one important paper (the van Buchem paper in the *British Medical Journal*) that the manual search turned up.

As always, a compromise is available. The Medline database is now available on compact discs. Using these along with suitable equipment and a personal computer allows for a far quicker search—more limited in scope than the traditional computer search, but potentially better than a manual search. As more libraries have this facility it is possible to sit at the computer desk and scan thousands of references with the press of a few buttons.

EXERCISE 1.4

If you have not already done so, take the opportunity of visiting your local postgraduate centre library and introducing yourself to the librarian(s). Discuss with them how you should set about answering the question of whether antibiotics are of value in the treatment of otitis media.

Search the literature, either manually, electronically, or both, to find which papers have been published in the last year in English language journals on two of the following:

1. a subject of your own choice
2. the treatment of anxiety in general practice
3. screening for glaucoma
4. the use of practice nurses
5. patient access to their own medical records.

Searching, by whichever method you choose, should allow you to see if there already exists an answer to a question that has entered your mind. Colleagues, textbooks, specialists, and even original papers must be carefully scrutinized and critically evaluated before deciding that your particular question has been insufficiently investigated.

QUESTION 1.4

Take a few minutes before finishing this chapter to note down your answers to the following:

1. What are the benefits from *my* doing research?
2. What stops *me* doing research?

(IT'S EASIER THAN YOU THINK)

There are many reasons why people undertake research. Some feel it necessary to continually question established practices, others see it almost as a means of confirming their faith in an organized, rational world of cause and effect. Again it might be seen as a challenge, a form of intellectual nourishment. Obviously there are some who do it just for fun, or to give a wider horizon to the daily work they do. It could also be thought by some to be a form of self-discipline needed to improve personal performance—or that the nature of experiment will help develop powers of imagination and critical sense. Of course, most do it for the thought of fame, fortune, and foreign travel. Although fortune is extremely unlikely there is a great deal of personal satisfaction to be gained from the development of a question into a research project leading to the production of a paper and its publication in a recognized medical or scientific journal—hardly fame, but much pleasure. And while there is no guarantee of foreign travel you will at least get out to visit your local postgraduate centre. Why then do more people not do research?

Can it be that they are all too lazy or apathetic? Is it just that they lack research skills and knowledge of research methods? Is it that research is considered irrelevant to daily life—a thing apart, to satisfy the egos of those who indulge in it?

If a major stumbling block is indeed the lack of research skills, or even a fundamental disbelief in the research method as a means of developing understanding, then perhaps it would be helpful to examine similarities between the research method and the clinical method taught in medical schools and still almost universally used when doctors see patients.

Let us consider similarities between the two methods:

Research method	Clinical method
• problems identified	• problem identified (through patient's complaint)
• formulating hypotheses	• hypothesis formulation to explain observations (differential diagnosis)
• testing hypotheses	• testing (examination of patient, other investigations, effect of treatments)
• conclusions	• conclusions (diagnosis)
	• follow-up.

There are strong similarities between the clinical method as used every day and the research method. The patient presents facts to the doctor ('the presenting complaint'). Almost immediately the doctor begins to arrange these facts in his or her mind, and starts to construct hypotheses to explain these facts. Testing takes place by asking more direct questions ('History of the presenting condition').

Patient: Doctor, I've had this pain in my chest for a couple of weeks
(Hypotheses: This pain could be cardiac in origin. This pain could be muscular. This pain could be pleuritic. This pain could be anxiety… and so on.)

Doctor: When does it tend to occur?'
(Testing several loose hypotheses at once.)

Patient: Mainly at night when I lie down.
   (Conclusion—less likely to be cardiac.)
   (Hypothesis: This pain could be reflux oesophagitis.)

Doctor: Does it occur at any other time—with food, coughing, bending over, for example?
   (Testing new hypothesis as well as others.)

The verbal examination will produce a set of hypotheses that are tested by the physical examination, then redefined or reconstructed and perhaps retested by the ordering of special investigations (e.g. in this example, chest X-ray, ECG, barium swallow, and so on) and possibly by the prescribing of a specific remedy (antacid, for example). A conclusion is then reached after a period of time (which in itself is often an important test of some hypotheses in general practice), as to whether one of the hypotheses has been sufficiently supported. If the conclusion is that it has not, then the process begins again.

And despite what would appear to be a fairly marked 'similarity' between the research method and the clinical method, GPs and consultants still shy away from doing research on the grounds of professed ignorance of its method!

SUMMARY

In this chapter we have looked at the meaning of research and how it could fit into the working pattern of every thinking health-care professional. We have explored the different types of questions that can be asked and how they might be sifted. Finally, ways to check to what extent the answer is known have been described.

SUGGESTED TASKS

1. Research can be an isolated business. Try and find out what local research facilities and support are available. Is there a local university or college with skills which you might call upon for help and advice?
2. Is there any research actually going on locally? Try asking the following:

- the FHSA
- the local Health Authority
- the LMC
- trainer workshops and young principal's groups.

3. Persuade some other GPs each to bring six possible research questions to a meeting at which their feasibility and interest would be evaluated.

ANSWERS TO EXERCISES

EXERCISE 1.2

1. No—tautologous question. Diabetes is defined in terms of raised fasting blood sugars.

2. Yes—answer is not immediately apparent, although may exist within the literature. The question *is* important, the prescribing of NSAIs is common, and the question has obvious general application.

3. Yes—again the question concerns a common area of concern, has a general application and is testable.

4. No—the question is important, is testable, but is of little general application. However, within this constraint the balance may still lead one to want to answer the question as it stands—so the answer could be 'yes'.

5. No—the arguments are the same as the previous question—possibly important, possibly testable but of no general application.

6. Yes—the question concerns a common condition, is testable, has general application, and obviously may lead onto further questions.

EXERCISE 1.3

Questions 1, 3, and 5 are more like audit questions in that they involve comparing against a standard (whether explicit or implicit): they all have the assumption that something is 'wrong' if the standard is not being met. Questions 2 and 4 are basic research questions.

2 Designing a study

Chapter 1 looked at the types of research questions that can be asked, and at ways to check to what extent the answer was known. Once the research question(s) has been chosen, the next step is to identify the design that will be appropriate for answering it. Let us work through an example showing how different types of research design can be devised for different types of question.

Most GPs are committed to reducing smoking among their patients. Dr Philip Tipps is aware that the local health promotion department is about to introduce an anti-smoking campaign, and he would like to see the effect of this on his practice population.

Question 1. Does the anti-smoking campaign reduce smoking in the practice population?

The question seems well-defined, fairly specific, and, above all, answerable. The next step is to devise a blueprint for how the question(s) will be answered—what is called the research design.

WHAT IS THE RESEARCH DESIGN?

The research *question* is expressed in ideas and concepts, whereas the research *design* is the plan of how the research will be carried out. It tends not to deal with specifics, but rather addresses the broad strategy of how the research will seek to answer the question. Getting the research design right is very important:

- it must enable the question to be answered; get it wrong and no matter what follows the results will not be able to answer the question
- it must also try to rule out 'alternative answers' to the research question.

It is at this stage that you might find that what were apparently 'answerable' questions are in fact unanswerable because a practical research design cannot be devised within existing resource constraints. Ideally the design should be chosen to fit with the research question, but in practice it is sometimes necessary to amend the question to fit in with the feasibility of the research design. This revision of research questions, sometimes as a result of other influences such as the knowledge gained through the literature review, is acceptable as long as the original problem is not entirely lost sight of.

In thinking through the best design for the question (Does the anti-smoking campaign reduce smoking in the practice population?) it is apparent that it can be expanded into three separate questions:

Question 1. What is the proportion of smokers in the patient population before the campaign?
Question 2. What is the proportion of smokers in the patient population after the campaign?
Question 3. Is the second proportion less than the first?

In summary, the research question has told Dr Tipps that the design required should provide a descriptive profile of one characteristic of the behaviour of a defined patient population both before and after the intervention.
Let's look at certain aspects of the research design in turn.

What is the population?

In principle the question is answered by asking all patients if they smoke or not. But how can Dr Tipps get hold of 'all patients'? They are never all collected together in one place. Various lists of all patients are available, so instead of collecting them physically together Dr Tipps can write to each individually and collect all their replies.

QUESTION 2.1

Dr Tipps would like to know which of his patients smoke. In order to look at this problem he must first define who are his patients. He decides that he has three sources or sampling frames for such a list:

• the medical record envelopes
• the age–sex register his keen trainee insisted on two years ago, and untouched since
• the FHSA register.

What are the advantages and disadvantages of each?

• Obviously the record envelopes are unwieldy, are arranged alphabetically, and probably contain many records of patients who have either died, moved, or been transferred, or they may be lying in the back of a partner's car (the records that is, not the patients).
• His own age–sex register has lain undisturbed for two years, and although it is much more convenient to handle, and is arranged chronologically, it will be grossly inaccurate by now. Even age–sex registers in well-organized practices have been found to be 5–10 per cent inaccurate when checked against FHSA registers.
• The FHSA may be able to provide the most up-to-date list of patients, but this again will be subject to significant inflation due to the problem of belated and slow withdrawal of patients—again evidence suggests around 10 per cent inaccuracy in FHSA lists.

EXERCISE 2.1

If Dr Tipps had wanted to extend his survey to include the whole population of the small town in which his was one of four practices, where might he have been able to obtain his population list?

Three common sources are:

- telephone directory
- electoral register
- Council tax records (for households rather than individuals).

What do you think might be the problems in using each?

Suggested answers can be found at the end of the chapter.

Which patients smoke?

Having established who are the population, the next stage is to separate smokers from non-smokers. Had Dr Tipps been using his medical record cards as his population list he could have checked through them to identify smoking habits—though it is doubtful if smoking behaviour would have been recorded in all or indeed many of them. If the information is not already available he will have to collect it anew.

He could send out a letter to all of his patients. This would give him the 'best' result, if they all replied. However, research is not only about getting valid results; it is also about being efficient in the light of the original question. The question is about a proportion who smoke, not about whether or not a particular patient smokes. It is therefore not necessary to ask every patient, but instead to ask a group of typical patients: if they are typical then their responses should be similar to those of other patients who are not asked. In other words, the solution is to ask a *representative sample* of the total population if they smoke. So long as the sample is truly representative, in other words it has identical characteristics to that of the total population, then one can reasonably generalize from the results of that sample to the whole population: what is true for the sample should be true for the population.

The advantages of using a sample are:

- it is more efficient in that it generally saves money, labour, and time
- with fewer cases it is easier to collect and deal with more detailed information from each case.

On these grounds, Dr Tipps decides to select a sample. But how does he do this? The next section will examine sampling in some detail before returning to the research questions on smoking.

SAMPLING

There are various types of sample. At the end of this chapter you should know the difference between some important samples, namely *random*, *systematic*, *stratified*, and *quota*.

QUESTION 2.2

Dr Tipps fortunately discovers that his practice manager has recently updated and corrected his age–sex register in line with the list held by the FHSA. This is held on the Royal College of General Practitioners' age–sex cards in two tin files, one containing all the males, the other all the females.

He decides to use these patient lists as the source from which to draw his sample, and therefore one weekend he takes the two tins home. A count of the cards reveals that he has 1200 male and 1300 female patients. He decides to take a 10 per cent sample of the patients aged 16 and over, which works out at 85 men and 95 women.

The method he first chooses is to close his eyes and extract 85 consecutive cards from the middle of the male tin, and 95 from the middle of the female tin.

What might be the problem, or biases, introduced by this method?

From the middle of the male tin the first eight cards he might pick out are:

John MacEwan
Angus McTavish
James McTavish
Robert McTavish
Fred McTell
Brian Niall
George O'Connor
Patrick O'Malley.

Dr Tipps begins to realize that names can cluster into ethnic and family groups.

Selection using this method is quite easy and convenient, but it does not meet the requirement for the research question to give a true cross-section of the patient population. This sample is unlikely to be sufficiently similar to the total population to enable him to generalize because it is not being selected from the whole patient population and every patient has not got an equal chance of selection. It is a sample of sorts but it is not a *representative sample*.

How can you ensure a representative sample?

For a study that measures the proportion of patients who smoke, Dr Tipps needs a sample that reproduces as accurately as possible the characteristics and qualities of the population on his list (which is the population he is studying). The intention is to use the results from the sample not just to draw implications for the sample itself but also to discuss the implications for the total population.

Random sampling is the most popular method for attempting to select a representative sample because it ensures that each person in the population has an equal chance of being selected.

QUESTION 2.3

Dr Tipps decides that his sample drawn as a group from his tins is not sufficiently representative of the population he wishes to study, for the reasons given above.

He decides to select every tenth card from each tin starting with those aged 16 and working upwards through the age groups. Has this overcome all the objections with his previous method? Is this a truly random sample?

Well, it is definitely better than the last sample, but it is not strictly speaking a random sample, unless the age–sex cards had all been filed in a random order. (And since this defeats the object of an age–sex register it is unlikely to be the case.) This type of identification of one sample member whose selection is dependent on the selection of a previous one is called a *systematic sample*. In a small sample it will tend to produce a more even spread over the population list than does a simple random sample. In this instance a systematic sample is probably acceptable as it is unlikely that there is any constant 'pattern' in the ordering of patients. Selecting every thirteenth playing card from an unshuffled new pack would of course produce a very unrepresentative sample.

Undeterred, Phil decides he really wants a truly random sample, and so decides to use a table of random numbers (having discovered that this can be found in the back of many statistics books). In the table he uses he finds that, starting at the top left corner, he must select the 3rd, 47th, 43rd, ..., notes in turn, using a table of random numbers like the following:

03	47	43	73	86	36	96	47	36	61
97	74	24	67	62	42	81	14	57	20
16	76	62	27	66	56	50	26	71	07
12	56	85	99	26	etc.				

Alternatively he could have used some form of lottery, drawing the patient numbers out in a version of research worker's bingo. He could even have emptied the cards on his living room floor, mixed them all up thoroughly and trained his pet woodpecker, Woody, to pick out the required number. For obvious reasons, or since Woody was off-colour, he decided to use the tables of random numbers.

How big should the random sample be?

Should Dr Tipps select one patient in five, one in ten, or one in how many? The rule of thumb, given that many studies have severe practical limitations on them, is the bigger the better. However, it is no good selecting a large sample if there are no facilities to gather or cope with the data when collected, nor a small one if it will not produce a valid result.

However, it is possible to calculate an idea of sample size required, by using some statistical techniques. The methods and the exact formulae used will vary with the type of question being asked and the thing being measured but they are based on the same principles. The use of statistics in research projects will be looked at in a later chapter but their use in relation to sample size will be outlined now. (Don't worry if you don't follow the steps completely. You can always return to this later, especially when you have a practical problem of deciding on a sample size for your own study; besides, by then you may have discovered the sample size calculator in the Epi Info program (see Chapter 8) or found a helpful local statistician to do the calculation for you.)

Dr Tipps wishes to know the proportion of his practice population over 16 who smoke. Let us assume the true figure is actually 34.5 per cent.

If he were to take, say, five randomly chosen samples of 100 patients over 16, and asked them whether or not they smoked, he might find the following results:

	Smokers	Non-smokers
Sample 1	35	65
Sample 2	36	64
Sample 3	40	60
Sample 4	17	83
Sample 5	33	67

It is obvious that most results cluster around what is actually the real population mean, but there are some outliers. If, by chance, sample 4 was drawn then an invalid result would be produced to the question, 'What proportion of patients smoke?'

What is clear is that if he took a very large number of samples, say 50 samples of 100 patients each, the mean of all of these 50 sets of results would to all intents and purposes equal the mean of the population from which he took the sample. Some of the results would exactly equal the mean, some would be slightly more, some slightly less, and a few would be considerably more and a few considerably less than the mean. A graph drawn of these sets of results would appear as in Fig. 2.1. The graph is roughly bell-shaped—the ubiquitous *normal* curve, of

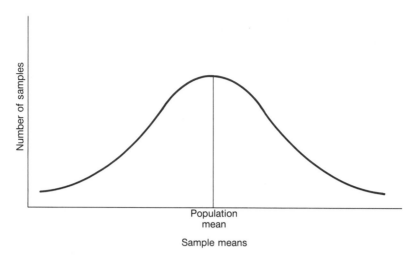

Fig. 2.1 Normal curve.

which doubtless you will have heard. In this normal curve derived from the means of a number of different samples:

• Most of the results will be clustered around the true mean of the population—hence the 'bell' shape of their distribution. The exact shape of this bell can vary, depending on how closely around the true mean value the results occur. A tall peaked bell suggests that all the results were bunched around the mean value, whereas a flatter-shaped bell suggests a wider spread of values.

• There is a number that describes and summarizes the spread of this distribution and which can be calculated: it is known as the *standard error of the mean*. This figure is useful as it is known that 95 per cent of the means of each of the 50 samples taken will fall within 1.96 standard error distances from the true mean. In other words, the means of between 47 and 48 of the separate samples can be expected to fall within the true population mean plus or minus 1.96 times the particular standard error of this population.

Why is all this important? Well, usually only one sample is taken—after all, the whole idea of sampling is to cut down on the amount of time and effort. There is therefore a need to have some idea of the shape of the curve to which the mean of this sample belongs (whether the 'bell' is likely to be peaked or flat), and as a consequence how likely is it that one sample mean is close to the true mean. In short, the standard error of the mean can be used to give an indication of how likely the mean of a single sample (and therefore the representativeness of the sample) approximates the mean of the whole population.

Because Dr Tipps wishes to know a proportion of a population with a certain characteristic, he can use the following formula:

$$\text{S.E.} = \sqrt{\frac{p(1-p)}{n}}$$

where S.E. is the standard error, p is the proportion of the population with the characteristic being measured (in this case smoking behaviour), n is the sample size, and the population is known to be very large with respect to the size of the sample taken.

Let us assume that Dr Tipps only took one sample, and it was in fact Sample 1 where he found that 35 per cent of the sample smoked: what could he say about the result with respect to his population? Using the formula above, the standard error of his one result can be found to be 4.77:

$$\text{S.E.} = \sqrt{\frac{35 \times (100 - 35)}{100}}$$

$$= 4.77.$$

This means that he can state that there was a 95 per cent chance that the true mean would fall within the range of the result found in this sample and 1.96 times the standard error: $35 \pm (1.96 \times 4.77)$. In other words, there is a 95 per cent likelihood that the true proportion of his population who smoke lies between 35 ± 9, i.e. between 26 and 44 per cent.

If his sample size had only been 10, the standard error would have been

$$\text{S.E.} = \sqrt{\frac{35 \times 65}{10}}$$

$$= 15.$$

In this case he would only have been able to say that there was a 95 per cent chance that the population mean was in the range $35 \pm (1.96 \times 15)$, that is between 6–64 per cent. As can be seen, the accuracy of the estimate for the population depends on the size of the sample. However, the extra accuracy to be gained by increasing the sample size tails off rapidly.

EXERCISE 2.2

What would be the effect if his sample size had been:

- 500
- 1000

(You may need a calculator for the sums.)

Answers are to be found at the end of the chapter.

At this stage Dr Tipps' interest lies in using the formula above to estimate the *size of sample* required. The above formula can be rewritten in terms of *n* (the required size of the sample) as

$$n = \frac{p\,(1\text{–}p)}{(\text{S.E.})^2}$$

It is unlikely that *p*, the proportion that smoke, and S.E., the standard error are known, so therefore estimates and judgements must be used. In particular:

- the proportion, *p*, must be found or guessed
- a decision has to be made about the size of the standard error—that is, how accurate the sample is required to be in terms of how large or small a spread of results around the true mean will be acceptable.

For example, before taking his one sample, Phil Tipps visits his local postgraduate library to look up the latest edition of *The general household survey*, an annual report from the Office of Population Censuses and Surveys based on a national sample of households. There he discovers—among data on the leisure activities and health habits of the population—that about 40 per cent of the national population are current smokers. He also decides that he would like the result to be within about 10 per cent of the true result, that is if the true result for his population is 36 per cent, he wants to be 95 per cent certain that the result from his sample falls in the range 36 ± 3.6 per cent. He also knows that 95 per cent of the samples will be within 1.96 standard errors of the mean. Therefore for his project he estimates that *p* will be 40 and that he needs the standard error to equal 1.8 (i.e. 3.6/1.96).

Substituting into the formula gives:

$$n = \frac{40 \times 60}{1.8 \times 1.8.}$$

This suggests that he requires a sample of around 750 to give him a result with the sort of accuracy he wishes.

As has been pointed out, the formula used above is only suitable when the characteristic being measured is a proportion. Other formulae based on exactly the same principles can be used for other measurements.

In the case of the simple question, 'What proportion of the practice population currently smoke?', the method is quite straightforward as the aim is to get a large enough sample to represent accurately the smoking behaviour of the background population. This accuracy then needs to be seen in the context of the possible change in smoking habit consequent to the health promotion campaign: if it is estimated that the campaign will reduce smoking by about 5 per cent then a sample size that is accurate only to about 10 per cent will clearly obscure any effects of the intervention. In this before-and-after design, the sample size calculation therefore needs to take account of the likely change brought about by the intervention and select a sample size that will allow such a change to be identified amidst the 'noise' caused by the sample mean being only approximate to the true population mean. Similar principles apply in the relevant calculation. Fortunately there are experts who will help you with these technical issues (and the computer program Epi Info, described in Chapter 8, can help with this problem).

Not being able to grasp the meaning of the standard error need not prevent you from carrying out excellent research. Besides, for a lot of research this is not an issue: you either collect a total population sample, such as all your asthmatics, or as many as you can within the limits of your resources. There are, as we shall see in later chapters, ways of handling imperfect samples. However, because a sample size is often not calculated, it does not mean that it is always superfluous. Had the researchers in many studies completed this simple calculation then their sample would have been seen as too small to obtain a significant result or—just as important—too large and therefore wasteful of time and resources.

EXERCISE 2.3

1. Dr. Tipps decides that he needs a more accurate result. He would like a 95 per cent chance of the result being within 3 per cent of the true mean. How large a sample would he need?
2. But this is the real world, he is a busy GP and he decides he can only afford the time to take a sample of 100. What predictions could he make about the accuracy of the result he will obtain from this sample in respect to the population?

Answers are to be found at the end of the chapter.

Dr Tipps decides on his sample size and picks the cards out of his age–sex tins at random. He is dismayed to find that by chance he has only picked out a small handful of teenagers, and he was particularly interested in the effect of the health promotion campaign on this group.

QUESTION 2.4

Our Dr Tipps decides that he wants to make sure that each age band, as well as each sex, is adequately yet randomly represented in his sample since he believes that one of the factors which is most strongly associated with smoking behaviour is age. How could he, with his age–sex register at home, allow for this.

Well, he has allowed for gender by selecting from his two separate tins; this ensures that men and women are fairly represented in the total sample. If he further wanted to ensure adequate representation of each age band he could 'group' his ages, as if in separate tins, before sampling from them. Thus first he could calculate the number of patients within each band, i.e. those aged 16 to 25, 26 to 35, 36 to 45, and so on, calculate the numbers required for his 10 per cent sample, and then, by using the table of random numbers, select an appropriate random sample from each of these age strata within each sex. This is a *stratified random sample*. In this case it would be stratified for age and sex.

For example, if Dr Tipps is particularly concerned about smoking among under 25s he may wish to stratify by age to ensure their adequate representation in the sample. First he calculates the number of 16–25 year-olds among men and women in the practice. Dr Tipps finds that this age group accounts for almost exactly 15 per cent of both men and women. If he used random sampling he would therefore expect to obtain 27 individuals from this group in his overall sample of 190 patients. However, he may, by chance, only get 24 or even 20 (though he may of course get more). By age stratifying his sample into under and over 25 he can then randomly choose 27 and 163 cases from each group, so ensuring correct representation of his under 25s.

Dr Tipps could also take this logic further. He might decide that 27 is rather a small group to analyse, particularly when split into men and women. He might therefore 'weight' his under 25 sample by a factor of, say, 4, thereby choosing 108 instead of 27 patients. He could always 'reconstitute' his original representative sample by dividing the under 25s by 4 and adding them back in.

In summary, stratification is the process of dividing the sample population into strata prior to sampling so as to increase precision and representativeness, especially of limited sample sizes. Usually factors chosen for stratification are those felt to be closely related to the subject of the survey, although selection of factors will also depend upon availability of information. For example, although social class is also likely to be strongly associated with cigarette smoking it may be impossible to stratify because there is unlikely to be information on social class in an age–sex register.

EXERCISE 2.4

1. You are concerned that some patients have difficulty in getting up the steep driveway to your surgery. You decide to find out who they are by means of a questionnaire. Who would you send it to?

1. a random sample of all your patients
2. a random sample of those attending this month
3. an age-stratified sample of all your patients
4. an age-stratified sample of patients who consult this month
5. all those who your receptionists note have had difficulty with the driveway.

2. You wonder if your patients would like to read their own notes. You design a questionnaire. Who would you send it to?

1. a random sample of all your patients
2. a random sample of all your patients over 16
3. a random sample of all your patients who can read
4. a random sample of all the patients who see you in the next week.
5. a random sample of your most responsible patients.

3. You wonder if the time you spend counselling your patients is having any effect. You decide to allocate randomly to a counselling and non-counselling group and count the number of subsequent consultations as a measure of success. Who would you enter into the study?

1. all the patients you see in a week
2. all the patients with psycho-social problems you see in a week
3. a random sample of all your patients
4. any patient you see with blue eyes
5. any patient you see with a birthday on an odd day of the month.

Suggested answers are to be found at the end of the chapter.

The first step of Dr Tipps' project, namely finding out what proportion of patients smoke, could count as a simple descriptive study in its own right. Answering the question 'How many?' can be important, especially in so-called prevalence studies which attempt to find the extent of a medical problem in the community, perhaps as the basis of making decisions on appropriate services. But Dr Tipps' project differs from a simple descriptive study in its attempt to explore the relationship between two phenomena, namely smoking and a health promotion intervention. Descriptive studies essentially look at one variable, depicting its size, extent, patterning, and so on. (How many cases of epilepsy are there in the community? How often do patients with diabetes consult in a year?) Two-variable studies tend towards explanation rather than description in examining a relationship. (Are men more likely to be epileptic? Is epilepsy related to un-employment?) Most commonly this explanation takes the form of exploring the extent to which one variable might cause another. The issue of causality and the related idea of correlation is central to most research studies.

• Does unemployment cause ill-health?
• Is sugar intake related to diabetes?
• Is asbestos linked with cancer?
• Does stress cause heart attacks?
• Is tennis playing correlated with baldness?

Each of these examples involves two variables held in some sort of relationship to one another: 'caused', 'linked', 'related', 'correlated', and so on. What do these words actually mean? They are all variations on 'cause', which is the fundamental link that any researcher is chasing, though some of them express the notion of cause in a very weak sort of way.

There are three conditions that must be fulfilled before it can be concluded that A, say, unemployment, causes B, say, ill-health:

• The temporal sequence must be right with A preceding B in time; that is the unemployment must precede the ill-health.
• There must be a correlation between the variables such that as A varies, B varies; thus unemployed people would be more likely to be ill compared with those in employment.
• There must be no significant 'third' variable or confounding factor which affects both A and B, such that the observed relationship might be 'spurious'; is it possible that those living in relative poverty are both more likely to become unemployed *and* get ill?

Let us look at this third condition in a little more detail.

All so-called causal relationships are in fact provisional and can be constantly subjected to challenge by suggesting other variables that explain the observed correlation. Thus for example the 'causal' connection:

$$\text{smoking} \quad \rightarrow \quad \text{IHD}$$

may really be:

$$\text{smoking} \qquad \text{IHD}$$
$$\nwarrow \qquad\qquad \nearrow$$
$$\text{tense people}$$

Thus, an important component of research is to take existing 'known' relationships that are believed to be causal and suggest alternative explanations of why the two (or more) variables seem to be related. Thinking of 'alternative explanations' is very important. Most 'great science' is not discovering new things but finding better explanations for known phenomena. Try it! When you are reading or listening to a research paper and you come across a supposed relationship between two or more variables think: how else might this relationship be explained? There are *always* alternatives; most are probably fanciful—cosmic rays, men from Mars, MI5 blunders—but occasionally you will come across an interesting alternative. The next stage is how to express this as a researchable question (back to Chapter 1), and then how to devise an appropriate design....

EXERCISE 2.5

Suggest some alternative hypotheses for the following supposed 'causal' relationships

1.	high blood sugar	retinopathy
2.	TB bacillus	tuberculosis
3.	smoking	gastric ulcer
4.	stress	ulcerative colitis
5.	promiscuity	cervical cancer
6.	snoring	CHD.

Suggested answers are to be found at the end of the chapter.

To continue with Dr Tipps' study of health promotion: what are the designs that might be available for assessing the impact of a stop-smoking campaign? In each case the design must enable the question to be answered and help rule out some of the more obvious alternative explanations. Let us explore a number of possible designs.

A simple design

The simplest design would involve collecting information from smokers *after* they had received advice from the health promotion campaign and comparing it with the rate beforehand. It would be useful to have 'baseline' data from a questionnaire before the intervention, but if respondents can be trusted to be truthful then only post-intervention data collection would be necessary. Let us assume that smoking declined: would that confirm the hypothesis that the campaign was effective? (in other words, is there an alternative explanation?)

Well, it is possible that something else happened at the same time (such as a tax increase on cigarettes) that produced the observed affect. It is important to allow for such extraneous factors—technically, *control* for them. But how can this happen without knowing what these factors are? The most straightforward way is to have a *control group* that will experience everything, including any other influences, except the health promotion campaign.

Use of a control group

The second design fulfils this condition in that it compares a group that did not receive the campaign with one that did. The two groups are then asked about their smoking practices over the last year or so. For example, if it is found that the 'campaign' group (the intervention group) reports a steeper decline in smoking than the control group, is it then possible to conclude that the advice is effective? A qualified yes, because there are still some caveats. The interpretation of the results depends on both how the two groups were selected and the reliability of retrospective reporting of smoking.

The selection of groups

The aim of the study design is to attempt to identify two groups identical in every way apart from the fact that one will receive the health promotion message and the other will not. Thus the method of selection of the two groups is crucial so as to minimize any bias.

Two methods are available:

- random allocation
- matched control groups.

Random allocation means that the group, intervention or control, to which a case is assigned for study is determined by chance, so that each case who enters the study has the same chance to be in either group. Thus, in the study of the effect of health promotion on cigarette smoking, each patient who is a current smoker could be randomly allocated using random numbers to the control or to the experimental groups (and then, perhaps, health promotion literature sent to the intervention group but not the control group). The concept of randomness was discussed briefly in the previous section and it will become clear that by using random allocation the two groups selected should be similar in terms of most characteristics, apart from the fact that one received advice and the other did not.

Matched control groups have certain similarities to stratified sampling in that some factors are deliberately manipulated rather than being left to chance as in randomization. Patients in the intervention and the control groups could be matched by factors such as age, social class, educational background, and other factors with which it is known that cigarette smoking varies, to ensure that both groups contain equal numbers of men, women, old, young, and so on.

One difficulty with matching is that it is not always clear which factors to match for; it may only be possible to match for some but not all the contaminating factors. A second problem is that if, say, five or six factors are being controlled for it may be difficult to find matching pairs. A simpler but less precise technique is to match the two groups for the variables separately, not in combination. In principle therefore, six middle-class married men and six working-class un-married men in the sample could be 'matched' by six working-class married men and six middle-class unmarried men in the control group—though in practice variables do get more mixed up than this.

Clearly if random allocation to the intervention and control groups were chosen it would have to take place prior to the campaign. If the study is a *retrospective* one, investigating the effect of an intervention that has already taken place—for example, comparing current respiratory illness in a group that did and did not receive antibiotics in childhood—then random allocation is impossible and the case control study comes into its own.

A *case control study* involves examining the effect of some intervention retrospectively through matched groups. Thus, it would be possible, after the health promotion campaign, to identify a group of patients who had stopped smoking and a group who had not, matched in other respects. The groups would then be compared to see how many had experienced the health promotion campaign. If significantly more in the stopped-smoking group had experienced the campaign than those in the continuing-to-smoke group, then it would be a reasonable conclusion that it was the campaign that had brought about the result.

Retrospective data

Because the research is concerned with possible causal influence of the campaign (the intervention variable) on cigarette smoking (the outcome variable), it would be helpful to have a design which:

- shows changes in smoking behaviour over time
- can identify the relationships between these changes and the advice given in the campaign.

The aim would be to compare changes in smoking during a time period starting sometime before and finishing some time after the campaign. This would also apply to the control group. However, in the case of the two-group design, reliance must be placed on smokers' reports of their current behaviour and their past behaviour gathered through information collected after the advice was given.

This gathering of data through retrospective reports is a popular method for trying to find out about changes over time and the factors that influence them. However, retrospective reporting is fraught with problems associated with:

- weakness in memory recall
- current experience and behaviour colouring reports of past behaviour
- reports influenced by what 'ought' to have occurred.

Each of these problems is important, although the first two could equally apply to both campaign and control groups. However, the third problem may apply particularly to the advice group who may tailor their reports of the degree of change of smoking behaviour to what they feel the doctor wanted to happen.

Before-and-after design

The third design overcomes the problem of retrospective reports and the inherent biases. This design is what is called a before-and-after design where the behaviour in question is measured both some time before and after the intervention. This before-and-after procedure would also have to be used in the control group or comparison group. This would ensure that changes in behaviour found to be associated with the intervention did not reflect changes in behaviour that had occurred concurrently, perhaps generated by other influences such as a national campaign aimed at changing smoking habits, or large increases in the price of cigarettes.

The idea of following up the same group (cohort) of people to identify changes in behaviour or other factors is described as a *cohort* or *longitudinal* design, in contrast to the measurement at one point in time which is called a *cross-sectional* design. Longitudinal designs involve returning to the respondents for further information in the future.

The best design to test the proposition, then, would be a two-group before-and-after design. This design can be refined in a number of different ways to cope with other issues. For example, if both groups were to be interviewed about their cigarette smoking before and after, there may be concern about the effect of the interview on behaviour. The interview may have the effect of raising awareness and encouraging modification in smoking behaviour. Thus, a third group would need to be added which not only did not receive the health promotion advice but also had a brief form to complete rather than an interviewer-administered questionnaire.

It should be clear from the above discussion that in general practice, choice of research design has to be pragmatic: there might be an 'ideal' design, but often practical constraints involve choosing another. This does not mean however that the more 'classical' formal research designs, as found for example in epidemiology, are not used in general practice; indeed, several of the more common ones have been covered above. These have included the use of experimental designs such as randomized or case control studies and longitudinal designs aimed at measuring changes over time.

EXERCISE 2.6

Identify the appropriate research *design* for answering the following questions:

1. Do men have higher consultation rates than women?
2. Do longer consultations increase levels of patient satisfaction?
3. Are working-class patients more likely to be dissatisfied with their doctors than middle-class patients?
4. What proportion of the patients on your list are heavy drinkers?
5. Do shorter consultations lead to higher prescribing rates?

Suggested answers are to be found at the end of the chapter.

The results of the study may show that the advice given in the health promotion campaign has had a major impact or perhaps only a modest one. But if it had no effect at all, or at least no measurable effect, another question arises:

Question 4. Why did the intervention have no effect?

This question is trying to investigate the relationship between variables, but not just in a statistical sense as it is concerned with understanding the *nature* of the relationship between the campaign and how the patient responded. It would seem better in this particular case to use a qualitative approach. If the research question starts with a 'why?' rather than a 'what?' or a 'how?', consider a qualitative study.

WHAT IS QUALITATIVE RESEARCH?

Quantitative research is concerned with counting, with reducing phenomena to number. But there are many phenomena, it is argued, that cannot be captured in a number, or at least are destroyed by any attempt to do so. Imagine you ask your patients how they feel today and one says 'I feel very grey today'. Perhaps that statement could be reduced to a number, but might it not be possible to keep and analyse the statement in its original form? This is the basis of qualitative research, which, as its name suggests, collects and analyses qualitative data.

One of the major criticisms levelled at much quantitative research is that it tends to restrict the sorts of answers that can be obtained. The question 'Have you come to the doctor today because you are ill, or because you want her to sign your passport form?' does not allow space for the patient who wants to catch up on last year's *Country Life* in the waiting room. The question 'Why have you come to the doctor today?' would pick this up, as well as a hundred other idiosyncratic reasons. Analysing these data is, as we shall see, difficult (the quantitative study's closed question is very straightforward in comparison), but at least it better captures the real reasons for attendance. This is why qualitative studies are often used to answer 'why' questions. The emphasis is on an intensive investigation of a small number of cases or settings. A qualitative approach can also be used in an exploratory way to establish the sorts of questions it would be most appropriate to ask in a quantitative questionnaire-based survey so that the possible answers provided for a question bear a closer relationship to respondents' real range of views.

A qualitative approach could be used in the investigation of why a health campaign about smoking is ineffective and could begin with interviews of a small group of smokers who received advice but did not report any change in behaviour. In this type of investigation the research design is of little importance as no claims are being made about the representativeness of the sample nor are attempts being made to control for extraneous factors. The emphasis is on understanding the nature of the relationship between variables and identifying the processes that shape that relationship. In this way, it might be found, perhaps, that the no-change group were not actually reached by the campaign, or interpreted the information about smoking in an idiosyncratic way, or did not seem to understand it.

One of the basic assumptions behind this type of interviewing is that people are not empty vessels but have their own complex belief systems supplied by their culture and influenced by their experiences. Thus any understanding of their behaviour and their reasons for their behaviour should begin by examining the sets of beliefs, rules, and meanings, that govern their daily lives. An understanding of smoking behaviour and the impact of health education advice will require an investigation of patients' beliefs about smoking, and its relationship to health and to the meaning of the advice received.

The methods adopted should aim to elicit the beliefs and feelings of the smoker without being influenced by the assumptions and values of the researcher. The most popular method for this approach is unstructured interviewing using tape-recorders. This involves the interviewer having a list of topics or general questions about which the interviewee is invited to express his or her own views. The tape-recorded interview is transcribed word-for-word and the transcripts are subsequently analysed (see Chapter 4 on data collection).

The method of sampling that could be used in this case would be *quota sampling*. Quota sampling makes no pretence at randomness; it simply means that the interviewer selects sufficient cases with the desired characteristics (women, elderly, bald men, ...) to make up the sample size. Because the emphasis is on examining the different types of relationships, it is important to choose, quite deliberately, a wide range of respondents. Quantitative studies tend to aim for typicality in their sampling, whereas qualitative research looks for heterogeneity.

The major weakness with quota sampling is that it is non-random and this makes it difficult, if not impossible, to estimate how representative the samples are of the population and this makes it of little value in quantitative studies. The major advantage of quota sampling is that it is economical and time-saving and is particularly useful in exploratory research using a qualitative methodology.

SUMMARY

In this chapter we have looked at the questions that need to be thought about when deciding on a research design for a study. Specifically, we have shown how the adoption of a certain type of design will depend upon the nature of the research question being examined.

SUGGESTED TASKS

Select some articles from medical journals and for each:

- identify the research question being asked
- identify the research design chosen
- think of alternative designs
- decide whether your alternatives would have been constrained on ethical grounds or by cost.

ANSWERS TO EXERCISES

EXERCISE 2.1

• The main advantage of the *telephone directory* is that it is easily accessible, though its major disadvantage is that it will be unrepresentative. While a majority of the population now have their own telephones, the proportion who do not will be mainly those who cannot afford to.

• An *electoral register* can be obtained from a public library. It is compiled every October and published the following spring. It lists, within each Polling District, all those entitled to vote (18 or over). It is probably the most convenient method for identifying a representative sample of the general population. The vast majority of people who are eligible to register actually do so (96 per cent), although it does not represent people under 18 and non-British subjects. There is also a problem with people who move (8 per cent per year) and how to trace them for interview.

• *Council tax records* have replaced rating and poll tax records. They can be obtained from local authorities (Valuation Officer). The major role of these records is to sample housing properties, in particular households living therein.

EXERCISE 2.2

• For a sample of 500

$$\text{S.E.} = \sqrt{\frac{35 \times 65}{500}}$$

$$= 2.1$$

Therefore the percentage of smokers was 95 per cent certain of being in the range 31–39 per cent, i.e. $(35 \pm (1.96 \times 2.1))$.

• For a sample of 1000

$$\text{S.E.} = \sqrt{\frac{35 \times 65}{1000}}$$

$$= 1.5$$

Therefore the percentage of smokers was 95 per cent certain of being in the range 32–38 per cent, i.e. $(35 \pm (1.96 \times 1.5))$.

As you can see, doubling the sample size when it already involves fairly large numbers has had a smaller effect on the precision of the answer obtained.

EXERCISE 2.3

1. Dr Tipps wants the answer to be more precise; he would like it to be within 3 per cent of the real value. He assumes again that the true mean is around 40 per cent, and therefore he would like to be 95 per cent certain that his result would be within 3 per cent of this, that is that the S.E. would be 3/1.96, or 1.5.

Substituting into the formula:

$$n = \frac{40\,(100 - 40)}{1.5 \times 1.5}$$

$$= 1067$$

Therefore in order to be 95 per cent certain that his result was within 3 per cent of the true mean, he would need to take a sample of about 1000.

2. He can only take a sample of 100. Again using his estimate of the result being around 40 per cent, he finds:

$$\text{S.E.}(p) = \sqrt{\frac{40\,(100 - 40)}{100}}$$

$$= 4.89$$

He therefore knows that the true proportion of smokers in his population is 95 per cent likely to be within 9.5 per cent of the mean he obtains from his sample.

EXERCISE 2.4

1.

1. This would work, but it is a big hammer to crack a small nut. Moreover, the numbers having difficulty with the driveway are likely to be small in the sample.

2. Some improvement on the above, at least you restrict it to those who consult; those who do not consult cannot have trouble with the driveway (unless they do not consult because they cannot make it up the drive).

3 and 4. Age stratification seems sensible: numbers having difficulty are likely to be few and more likely to be elderly so this, especially (4), should ensure that the main 'at risk' group is properly represented in your sample.

5. Why bother with the questionnaire? You could simply ask your receptionist. The problem is that your receptionist might miss some people—in which case a sample derived from them would be inappropriate.

2.

1, 2 and 3. These are all possibilities. Presumably you would want to restrict it to adults and to those who can read, but you are unlikely to have data on the latter. Thus sample (2) would seem the best of the three.

4. Consulters are not representative of all your patients, so this sample is 'biased'. However, it may be that the question of reading notes is more appropriate for consulters who might have both the wish and opportunity to read their notes. If you accept this assumption this would be the best sample.

5. Well, this is one way of fixing it. You could choose as 'responsible' all those patients who agree with your views; the result will then be to your liking. Politically shrewd—but is it research?

3.

1. This depends on whether you think counselling might benefit all your patients who consult. If you think it will, this would be the one to go for.

2. More realistically, you might want to start only with those who might be said to 'need' counselling.

3. But how can the non-consulters receive the treatment or non-treatment? You could use your total patient population to 'mark' out those who will and those who will not receive counselling if they do consult. If your question is truly random and your population large enough, you should have allocated those who consult with emotional problems next week into two equal-sized groups.

4. This is one way of getting a sample, but only 'safe' if blue eyes are totally unconnected to having emotional difficulties or being responsive to counselling. You probably cannot make these assumptions, particularly if your practice contains large ethnic groups.

5. Similar to (4), but less likely that birth date is related to illness or treatment. In fact this is probably a reasonable way of obtaining a 50 per cent sample or, by using odd and even birth dates, of randomizing patients between two groups.

EXERCISE 2.5

1. Arteriopathy might cause retinopathy and also affect the pancreas to interfere with insulin production, hence increasing blood sugar.

2. An 'autoimmune response' might generate a tuberculous-like lesion, e.g. Crohn's disease, and also allow the bacillus entry to the body if contact is made: hence they would tend to occur together as in gastro-intestinal tuberculosis.

3. Anxious people might be both more likely to smoke and more likely to get a gastric ulcer.

4. Stress may be a response in people genetically predisposed; they might also be genetically predisposed to ulcerative colitis. Hence the two would be more likely to occur together.

5. Women with unhappy childhoods might be more likely to be promiscuous; the unhappiness might also—through an unknown mechanism—make them more at risk for developing cervical cancer.

6. Impaired respiratory function might produce snoring as well as placing extra effort on the heart.

These are only suggestions—some of them fairly pathetic!—and you might have better ones. The important point to stress is the possibility of constantly searching for alternatives for both speculative and even 'established' truths.

EXERCISE 2.6

1. Cross-sectional surveys of representative samples drawn from both groups.

2. Cross-sectional survey of patients randomly allocated to receive long and short consultations.

3. Cross-sectional surveys of representative samples drawn from both groups; or case control study comparing, retrospectively, social classes of satisfied and dissatisfied groups.

4. Descriptive cross-sectional survey.

5. Same as (2).

3 Measuring things

This chapter describes how you will measure the things that you have decided need measuring from your research question and associated design.

PRELIMINARIES

In her clinical work Dr Melanie Warmhands has observed that relationships in the families of asthmatic children do not seem very good. How should she go about exploring this question? Let us briefly summarize the process covered so far.

First, as argued in Chapter 1, the hunch must be refined into a *researchable question*. This might be:

Question 1. The relationships between the parents of an asthmatic child are of poor quality.

Second, as presented in Chapter 2, an appropriate *research design* must be chosen for the project. In this case it must obviously involve examining the relationships between parents of asthmatic children to see if they are indeed of poor quality.

How will Dr Warmhands choose her sample?

QUESTION 3.1

Below are four different ways of getting a sample. Score each of these from 1 (worst) to 5 (best) for two qualities: ideal suitability and practical suitability.

A. Picking out the next 20 known asthmatic children who present
B. Questioning and examining all the children who present with asthma until there are 20 cases accumulated
C. Randomly selecting case notes of children until there are 20 with a history of asthma
D. Randomly selecting case notes of children, visiting them, and examining for asthma, until there are 20 cases.

Three of these methods of sampling have a bias, that is they involve selecting for criteria other than asthma:

Sample A is a selection of children

- with asthma
- who are attenders
- who are known to the GP.

Sample B is a selection of children

- with asthma
- who are attenders.

Sample C is a selection of children

- with asthma
- who are known to the GP.

Sample D is a selection of children

- with asthma (and open to bias in the representativeness of the case notes).

Should sample D therefore be chosen? There are other considerations, chief of which is practicality. Sample D is only obtained after considerable time and energy. In contrast, sample A, which is the most biased, is the most easily obtained. What relative weights should be give to these two factors of bias and practicality?

The answer has to involve consideration of the research question: if necessary it might have to be revised. The hypothesis as stated would suggest sample D is the best because the question tries to make a general statement about parents of *all* asthmatics. On the other hand, the question evolved from a clinical observation that presumably only involved known asthmatics and attenders. In this sense there is some justification in clarifying the research question:

Question 2. The relationships between the parents of known asthmatic children who consult their GP are of poor quality.

This hypothesis would allow the use of sample A; however, by narrowing the focus some other difficulties have been introduced:

- The research question is not as wide as it was, and it will not be possible to draw conclusions about non-attending asthmatics (though if the hypothesis was confirmed it would be possible to go on to spread the net wider in a follow-up study).
- The original question suggested some relationship between asthma in a child and parental dynamics, perhaps that poor parental relationships somehow 'pro-duced' asthma in their child. If a relationship between asthma and parental dynamics was found in this particular sample, a very plausible alternative explanation would have to be considered, namely that poor parental relation-ships cause attendance or cause their child to be brought for diagnosis. Some of this threat to the interpretation of the findings can be allowed for in the other important element of research design, namely a control group. In addition there is clearly a need for a control group to measure 'poor quality' because this obviously implies 'poorer quality than other parental relationships'. (If other

relationships are not checked it could be that all the parents on a GP's list have similar poor relationships and therefore asthma is not unusual in this respect.)

Dr Warmhands chooses sample A. She obtains 20 children for her sample. Which of the following would be a suitable control group?

- 20 other children seen in the period, randomly selected
- 20 other children seen in the period, with the same ages and sexes of the asthmatic sample, i.e matched
- 20 other children seen in the period, with chronic eczema.

Each of these control groups has its merits. A random sample, as in the first option, would go some way to allow for the characteristics of sample A that might otherwise confuse the answer to the question. Say, for example, that poor parental dynamics did not affect asthma but rather increased the likelihood of a surgery attendance; a relationship would then be found between asthmatics attending surgery and parental relationships because asthmatics also happen to be attenders. If there was a control group of random attenders these should also show poor parental relationships. Therefore it would be possible to conclude from this that the finding among the asthmatics was a *spurious* one, unrelated to asthma. On the other hand, if there was a difference between asthmatics and controls it would tend to support the view that it is the asthma itself which is the significant factor.

While a random sample has clear advantages as a control group, in practice quite large numbers might be necessary to be sure that extraneous factors have been properly randomized. For example, just by chance, the control group might have an average age higher than the asthmatic group, thus any observed difference in parental relationships might reflect this fact rather than the asthma. With small numbers, as in sample A, a matched control group removes some of the biases that might confound the comparisons. Thus matching for age and sex ensures that these factors cannot be used to explain any differences between the asthmatic children and the control group because they are both exactly the same with regard to these variables.

A control group with chronic eczema is another form of matching. Here the logic is to exclude factors from the study that might contaminate the role of asthma. Thus, it is possible that poor parental inter-relationship in asthmatics and attendance rates are somehow related, not to the asthma itself but simply to having a chronic illness. Hence by controlling for other chronic illnesses, or a specific one, any difference between the relationships in the two groups is more likely to be linked to asthma itself.

After due consideration of the above issues Dr Warmhands chooses this third control group. She now has a prospective matched control group design with which to test her hypothesis; now, on to measuring things.

MEASUREMENT: INSTRUMENTS AND OPERATIONALIZATION

In this study Dr Warmhands has to decide which attributes she is going to measure and what sort of 'ruler' she is going to use. The technical term for the device with which she will measure is an 'instrument'.

First, what does she need to measure? There would seem to be at least six different key words contained in the research question:

- children
- attendance
- asthma
- eczema
- parent
- interpersonal relationship
- other 'control' variables.

Each of these 'things' is a 'variable' because it can be expected to vary. In addition, they all have a certain abstract quality about them because at the moment they are simply words: it might be possible to guess what they mean, but for the research it is important to be very precise about how they are defined.

In technical terms each of these words is a *concept*. They are concepts because they involve an idea or quality that is fairly abstract. It is not possible physically to get hold of these qualities, though if it was known how to define or measure them then it should be possible to identify them. In short, what is needed is some measure or *indicator* of the concept. This process, of devising indicators for concepts, is known as *operationalization* and is the main concern of the rest of this chapter.

How does Dr Warmhands operationalize the variable list above? Let us take each in turn.

Children

It is generally understood what is meant by the word 'children', but for the moment suspend that knowledge while thinking through the process of how to measure 'children' in a research project.

It might be agreed that children are small, and playful, and lack the intellectual grasp of an adult. What rules can be derived from these ideas that would allow a person consulting to be assigned to the category child or not-child? There are various possibilities given the above ideas on what a child is:

- establish the person's height: those below 1.5 metres are children
- provide the person with coloured bricks and see if they play: if they do they are children
- establish their intellectual age: if it is less than 10 they are children
- ask their chronological age: if it is less than 12 they are children.

Which instrument is chosen will depend on what is meant by children *in the context of this study*. In a psychiatric study childlike intellectual activities might be sought in adults, but in this research there is a clear understanding that children are differentiated by their chronological age. This still leaves the cut-off point open. At what age does Dr Warmhands want children to be eligible to enter her sample, and at what age do they become too old? These decisions are fairly arbitrary. She decides that she is really only interested in asthma in school children and she therefore selects the ages of 5 and 15 as the bottom and top delimiters. Thus she concludes:

A child, in the context of this study, is anyone over the age of 4 and under the age of 16 at the time of being seen. Furthermore their quality of 'childness' will be measured by using a scale based on their age, i.e. from 5 to 15, which will be obtained by asking them how old they are.

Thus, on the one hand, she has clarified her concept from the rather broad 'children' to 'children aged 4–16 seen in surgery', and on the other, defined an indicator—a question on their age—with which to measure this concept.

The example of measuring what a child is may be somewhat trivial, but it illustrates both the logic of measurement and the fact that even very familiar things need to be clarified and defined *before* starting to collect data. In summary then, there is a *concept*, a child, which can be *operationalized* by using the response to the question 'How old are you?' as an *indicator*.

EXERCISE 3.1: CONCEPTS AND INDICATORS

Match the following *concepts* to their appropriate *indicators*.

Concepts	**Indicators**
income	aged over 65
elderly	presence of a vagina
women	sphygmomanometer reading
stress	monthly net salary
chronic illness	heart rate
GP workload	reported gender
referral rate	galvanic skin resistance
blood pressure	length of surgeries
	on disability register
	reports long-standing illness
	number of patients seen
	patients sent to outpatients

Suggested answers can be found at the end of the chapter.

You may notice that *taken in isolation* what is a concept and what is an indicator is rather arbitrary. Thus 'heart rate' is an indicator of 'stress', but equally heart rate could be treated as a concept and operationalized as, say, pulse rate in the radial artery. The key difference between the two is therefore their relative positions:

- concepts are always more abstract than indicators, indicators more empirical than concepts
- concepts are drawn from the hypothesis, indicators describe practical measurement procedures.

EXERCISE 3:2

Operationalize the following hypotheses:

1. older people are more likely to be diabetic
2. your concentration tends to lapse towards the end of a surgery
3. you have more elderly patients on your list than your partners
4. patients with stress in their lives consult more frequently
5. a patient's hand movement while describing an anginal pain is very characteristic.

Remember: If you wish, you could plan a research design for each hypothesis. In addition you should list the concepts you wish to measure and against each list one or more possible indicators.

> Suggested answers are to be found at the end of the chapter.

RELIABILITY AND VALIDITY

The instrument chosen to measure whether or not the patient is a child or not is basically the question 'How old are you?' The answer identifies whether or not this is a child for the purposes of the study and what 'childness' qualities they have. Having operationalized 'child' there are two important questions that need to be asked of the instrument:

- is it reliable?
- is it valid?

Reliability

Reliability is a technical term. It refers to whether or not an instrument gives consistent results. A ruler is reliable because successive measurements of the same length of string would produce the same result. Is the question 'How old are you?' reliable? Yes. It is highly unlikely that people's response will vary over a period of time (unless they have had a birthday). It may however be unreliable if applied to very small children, or in a pre-literate society in which chronological age is simply a guess.

Validity

Validity refers to whether the instrument measures what it purports to measure. A way of measuring may be reliable yet still be invalid; thus while readings from a sphygmomanometer may be consistent, they may be mistakenly consistent if the machine is miscalibrated.

For the moment there is a need to establish how valid the question 'How old are you?' is, as a means of measuring the chronological age of the child.

There are various different ways of establishing the validity of an instrument: the most basic are face validity and convergent validity.

Face validity

It can be argued that the instrument, 'How old are you?', is valid because it seems obvious that this question will establish a correct answer. This form of validity is referred to as *face validity* or *logical validity* because 'on the face of it' it seems correct.

Much of measurement in medicine relies on face validity. There is often a general consensus that certain 'instruments' actually measure what they purport to measure (hence the synonymous term of *consensus validity*). Thus, in clinical practice a high blood sugar indicates diabetes, raised cardiac enzymes a myocardial infarction, pain in the right iliac fossa appendicitis, and so on. And of course the same thing goes for research when measurement often seems uncontroversial.

The problem with this approach is that the instrument may be invalid, or a better one may be overlooked. Exacerbation of abdominal pain on walking is, for example, probably a better indicator of appendicitis than localization to the right iliac fossa (according to researchers who have studied the validity of various indicators of appendicitis). This does not mean that face validity is an unsuitable way of assessing the value of an indicator; in many situations it will be quite appropriate. But face validity is only one way of doing it, and a fairly primitive way at that, and alternatives need to be considered; above all you need to be aware of the assumptions behind face validity if you use it as the basis of your measurement.

Convergent validity

Face validity is in many ways the weakest way of establishing validity because it is clearly open to the idiosyncrasies of the researcher to decide what is 'obvious'. Perhaps children lie about their age? How can it be established that a question on their age gives a truthful answer? The simplest means is to seek corroboration: ask to see their birth certificate, check their notes, ask their parents. Again, at no point is there certainty, but if all these indicators provide exactly the same answer then there can be increased confidence that the initial instrument, namely a question to the child, is valid. It is exactly the same mechanism at work in diagnosis when two indicators of the disease—chest pain and ECG changes—mutually support the diagnosis.

This form of corroboration is called *convergent validity* in that different measures all 'converge' to support one another. In addition convergent validity can be divided into two types: *concurrent* in which the corroborative measure is established at the same time, or *predictive* in which the supporting data is gathered sometime in the future.

The surgeon usually looks for additional indicators of appendicitis beyond pain in the right iliac fossa before making the diagnosis; physicians will use an ECG recording to support the implications of raised cardiac enzymes. Does a high blood sugar indicate diabetes? Well, it might have predictive validity if it were established that patients with high blood sugar had a greater chance of developing retinopathy. And so on. In effect a disease or diagnostic category is simply a word given to a clustering of indicators.

EXERCISE 3.3

Professor Teasmade, the well-known GP and ornithologist, has just presented his latest research to a typically uncritical and ingratiating group of acolytes. Alert to the problem of the validity of his measures—and anxious to establish your reputation as a fast young blade—you publicly challenge him: what type of validity does he use in his replies?

Question 1. How do you know you measured blood pressure accurately?
Answer. My sphygmomanometer is recalibrated every six months.

Question 2. How do you know patients' self-reporting was a valid measure of chronic illness?
Answer. Because I checked them with my own impeccable clinical records.

Question 3. How do you know that you were able to distinguish severe angina from your series of chest pains?
Answer. Most of them had admissions for myocardial infarction the following year—that's pretty serious! (Laughter.)

Question 4. How do you know that you did not forget to record any patients when you calculated your consultation rate?
Answer. Because my devoted receptionist also kept a record.

Question 5. How did you establish which of your patients had a high stress level? (Cries of 'sit down!'.)
Answer. It was fairly obvious to a person of my skill and experience. (Applause.)

Suggested answers are to be found at the end of the chapter.

Attendance

The hypothesis requires the sample to be drawn from children who see the doctor. How is Dr Warmhands to accomplish this? Again, it is partly a definitional exercise because as long as attendance is defined and measured the same way for both asthmatic children and controls then they should be comparable. Even so, defining 'attendance' is not as easy as it might at first seem.

QUESTION 3.2

Which of the following children would be eligible for inclusion in a sample of *attenders*?
An asthmatic child:

* who is brought in with a cough
* who accompanies its mother who has booked the consultation for herself
* who comes to collect a repeat prescription for his or her parent
* whom you visit at home with abdominal pain
* whom you chance to meet in the local supermarket
* whom you visit in hospital following emergency admission.

There are in fact no right or wrong answers. The operationalization of 'attendance' can be fairly arbitrary so long as it is consistent. Thus Dr Warmhands might decide that:

Attendance is a consultation with the child in the surgery.

Is it reliable? So long as the decision is consistent. Is it valid? The indicator has face validity.

Asthma

How will asthma be measured? Dr Warmhands cannot, as in 'attendance'—and like Humpty Dumpty—say asthma is what she says it is, because there are accepted outside definitions of asthma that must act as her standard.

What is asthma? How is it defined clinically? A search of the literature will reveal that there is no generally accepted standard diagnostic criterion which can simply be taken off the shelf. There are many ways of defining asthma, and as many controversies about what exactly it is. How should Dr Warmhands go about choosing?

She could go back to the original clinical observation. What was meant by asthma in that observation? Can it be reproduced in a reliable way? Alternatively she could look to other researchers who have operationalized it and use their approach. What about taking reduced peak flow as an indicator?

• Is it practical/easy? Yes, it is a simple, cheap and straightforward technique that should be easy to carry out for 5 to 15 year olds.
• Is it reliable? There may be an existing literature on this that could be checked. Alternatively she could try it herself—clinically she may already be doing so by making three measures and choosing the 'best'. For research purposes, however, the interest is in the relative similarities of the readings. If, after an initial practice, readings seem reasonably consistent it can be concluded that the technique is reliable.
• Is it valid? Does a low peak flow indicate asthma? This is a question with several answers. First, it could be that a definition of asthma will include low peak flow. Second, there may already be a literature on the validity of peak flow as an indicator of asthma. Third, Dr Warmhands could herself try and establish, through convergent validity, the value of peak flow as a measure of asthma. What factors should correlate? A history of wheezing? Expiratory wheezes heard with the stethoscope?

In addition she might consider if there are other diseases that may produce a lowered peak flow and try and introduce a question or test to distinguish them from asthma. This might be termed *divergent* or *discriminant* validity.

Basically then there can be two different ways of measuring asthma:

• There might be a single indicator, say peak flow, which is known from corroborative evidence to identify asthmatics. The peak flow meter reading therefore becomes the criterion that could be adopted.
• It may be decided that asthma requires more than one indicator because either peak flow readings miss some cases or also include other diseases. Asthma might then be said to exist if the following conditions are met:

• there is a peak flow reading below a specified level
• there is a history of wheezing
• the stethoscope reveals bronchial wheezes.

Eczema

The control group of eczematous children poses similar problems of definition. What is to count as eczema and how severe does it have to be before it can be considered an appropriate control for asthma? Again recourse to a dermatology textbook or previous research on eczema may provide useful criteria for deciding what is eczema and what is not, though there may be 'mixed' or unclear skin lesions that cannot be precisely diagnosed. In addition there is the problem of measuring severity. Eczema may be a 1 cm square patch on the back of a hand or it may cover a large surface of the body. If there is not a standard 'meter' with which to measure it, how can it be measured accurately?

First, Dr Warmhands needs to make a judgement as to whether or not eczema is present. Next, she must devise fairly precise rules for making a clinical judgement on its severity. Thus, she might say that the severity of eczema should be scored on a three-point scale:

1. mild, patient relatively unconcerned, no interference with their lives
2. moderate, covers some sensitive body areas, patient concerned, needs treatment
3. severe, widespread, incapacitating, topical steroids necessary to control.

Perhaps those scoring 2 or 3 on the scale could join the control group.

Is this measurement practical? Yes, it can be carried out easily during the consultation.

Is it reliable? Assuming the lesion remained constant over a couple of weeks, reliability of the measure could be tested by seeing if an assessment on one occasion agreed with assessment on another. In practice the disease is likely to change over time so such checks may be difficult. How else could the consistency of this particular measure be assessed?

If Dr Warmhands were clearly to describe the scale of mild, moderate, and severe to two of her partners she could ask them to score the same patients and then compare results. If the results are consistently the same then the instrument (in effect a GP applying the scale) is reliable.

She could go further and ask two local dermatologists to help with the study. Again she would have to spend time with them agreeing what is to count as eczema and how they will operate the severity scale. Then, each case could be scored by five people: Dr Warmhands, her two partners, and the two dermatologists. Each would score eczema present or absent and, if present, what degree of severity (1, 2, or 3).

In practice this would be a rather elaborate procedure just to establish a control group, but the principle of using separate raters is a useful one for measuring something rather nebulous. It could be used, for example, in scoring a patient's quality of life if several raters all listen to a tape recording of a patient describing their life. There is a special term, 'inter-rater reliability', that describes the degree of agreement between different raters. These techniques will be covered in more depth in later chapters.

For the present it is sufficient to know that comparison of trained raters can be used to test reliability. Perhaps the word *trained* should be emphasized because assessing reliability in this way does depend on all the raters working the same way and, in effect, being tantamount to the same instrument. Pause for a moment and consider what would happen if your partners and the friendly dermatologists had not been 'trained'? In such a case the different assessments of the eczema by all five observers would not give a measure of reliability but of convergent validity: if, independently, they all agree on cases of, say, severe eczema then clearly their assessments are valid.

In summary, two *similar* measurements of the same phenomenon can be used to assess reliability; two *different* measurements, convergent validity. Difficulty can arise if it is not clear whether two measures are sufficiently similar (to assess reliability) or sufficiently dissimilar (to assess validity). Is the training of dermatology colleagues sufficient? If it is, they can help you assess reliability. If it is not, then they can help you establish validity.

Parent

The term 'parent' would again be operationalized in the light of the hypothesis. In a genetic study, parent no doubt would imply biological parent; in this study Dr Warmhands presumably means whoever is responsible for 'parenting' the child. In addition, she is looking for a relationship between parents so she needs two of them.

Thus she might define parents as a man and woman who have been looking after the child, as parents, during the last three years. This could be established from asking the 'parents' who accompany the child or the child itself. Reliability is likely to be high, and face validity is probably sufficient here.

Interpersonal relationship

Concepts such as child, parent, or attendance are relatively easy to operationalize: first they are fairly low-level concepts—they almost define themselves—so face validity is good, and second there is a good degree of consensus as to what the terms mean anyway. With concepts such as the quality of interpersonal relationships there are greater problems: the concept is very abstract so operationalizing can be difficult, and because the exact meaning of the term is not clear there are likely to be as many indicators as there are meanings.

What are the sorts of ways in which something as abstract as quality of interpersonal relationships can be measured?

Most measurement in medicine concerns physical things—bodies, diseases, biological parameters, and so on—and these can seem easier to measure than psychosocial parameters because they can somehow be 'seen'. But this view is rather simplistic. Blood pressure might be biological/physical, but in fact it cannot be seen. Clinicians put a device, the sphygmomanometer, between themselves and the blood pressure to make it visible. This is precisely the process described above whereby concepts are operationalized as indicators, so achieving practical ways in which they can be measured.

The measurement of social relationships can be approached in exactly the same way. Leaving aside for the moment the possibility of actually observing the relationship, how can Dr Warmhands transform the relationship as it exists in the parents' heads to an indicator that will express the relationship as a number, just as the sphygmomanometer translates the concept of blood pressure into so many millimetres of mercury? These principles are important because they can be used to transform any mental state—anxiety, depression, satisfaction, joy—into numbers that can then be used in research. Let us take the problem of how to convert thoughts into numbers; specifically, how can the views of a parent on the quality of the relationship they have with their spouse be rendered into some sort of numerical scale.

First, proceed as in the physical sciences: there is a phenomenon Dr Warmhands wishes to measure, therefore she has to devise an appropriate instrument (through operationalizing the concept), and then go ahead and measure it. A very simple instrument might be the question:

Question 1. Do you have a good marriage?

There are, as you might guess, some difficulties with this approach which do not occur for the natural scientist.

The problem of meaning

Measuring the length of several pencils is straightforward, because the characteristic 'length ' is constant in each pencil and between different pencils. With human beings, however, the object under study is not a passive constant: people are constantly changing and, moreover, they evaluate stimuli before reacting to them. In other words, before replying to a question, people inevitably evaluate the question ('What does it mean?') before replying. The pencil is not aware of the presence or intentions of the ruler, whereas people are aware of the presence of the researcher's instrument and infer intentions in the researcher. Thus, if someone believes the mark of a good marriage is to have lots of children their response to the question will, unknown to the researcher, be misleading.

Dr Warmhands therefore needs to develop some special techniques to try and manage this problem of meaning. It might be pointed out at this stage that some social researchers have argued that this problem is insuperable and that such research is always flawed. They would be more inclined to adopt the qualitative methods outlined in the previous and later chapters.

In essence, the problem of meaning potentially interferes with the validity of the chosen instrument as Dr Warmhands may not be measuring the phenomenon she thinks she is measuring; instead, she may be picking up her respondents' own idiosyncratic interpretations of her instrument. She therefore has to be very careful about the process of operationalization and the checks on validity. Let us go through the process step by step.

Concept: 'quality of a relationship'
(thinks: what does this actually mean....?)
...... operationalize......
Indicator: 'Do you have a good marriage?'

This indicator has face validity, but it has limitations:

• It is open to the patient's own interpretation of what is actually meant by the word 'good'.
• It is a rather narrow operationalization: in the initial hypothesis the quality of a relationship implied something much wider; in fact it might be argued that

despite starting with a multidimensional concept a unidimensional indicator was produced, a bit like measuring a box by only one of its three dimensions.

The question can be improved by replacing it with a question that is more focused; in addition, given that the concept is multidimensional, it might be sensible to try more than one question to tap different facets of the quality of a marriage. Try:

Question 2. Do you often have rows?
Question 3. If you have a problem can you talk it over with your partner?

Together these two questions constitute a very elementary questionnaire. How has Dr Warmhands improved on the first instrument?

• Because of patient interpretation of Question 1, it seemed likely to give an invalid result. Questions 2 and 3 are more focused and perhaps less subject to interpretation problems.
• This seems to be a better operationalization than Question 1. Already she is beginning to tap two important features of a relationship: does it suffer from breakdowns and is it generally supportive?

Of course she could go on adding questions to her questionnaire, each one tapping a different facet of what the researcher thinks might be the quality of the relationship. In principle the more questions, the better the questionnaire, but as will be discussed in Chapter 4 there are some practical constraints.

For the moment Dr Warmhands decides to stop at her two-question—or, as it is often called, two-*item*— questionnaire. She tries it out by asking one patient's parent 'Do you often have rows?', and they reply 'Not particularly'. Whatever does this mean? The problem of meaning can be seen to be a two-way phenomenon: the respondent must interpret the researcher's question and the researcher must in turn interpret the answer.

A series of patients might provide a series of answers to Question 1. 'Not particularly', 'Yes', 'Never, except over money', 'Less than might be expected', and so on. Dr Warmhands obviously needs to ensure that the responses she elicits make sense in terms of some sort of scale. The commonest way of achieving this is to provide a series of set answers and ask the respondent to choose the one closest to their answer. Thus she might have:

Question 4. Do you often have rows?   Yes ❏
                                                         No   ❏

(Please tick the appropriate box)

The difficulty with constraining respondents in this way is that in trying to avoid ambiguous answers she has imposed her own measuring system. Perhaps the respondent has rows twice a year: is that to count as 'often'? What exactly is meant by 'rows' and by the adjective 'often'?

In effect, there are two broad possible strategies here: one can ask short questions that force responses into perhaps inappropriate categories, or invite the respondent simply to talk about their rows, record these on tape and count this as the data collection. Thus:

Question 5. Do you often have rows?   Yes ❏

                                                            No ❏

or

Question 6. Tell me about any rows you have?

(tape on ...)

These two approaches can be differentiated as *structured* and *unstructured*. The latter will require considerable analysis and 'structuring' *after* data collection—a topic to be covered in Chapter 6. For the moment let us stay with Dr Warmhand's structured questionnaire.

It is clear that the structured questionnaire and associated response frame she has devised above is very short and crude. How can it be improved?

She could, of course, add new questions to tap other aspects of the relationship, or indeed, further questions to clarify the questions already asked, such as exactly what is meant by rows. Perhaps:

Do you ever quarrel about money?

Do you have disagreements about child care?

Do you believe occasional arguments help to clear the air?

And so on.

In addition she can widen the response frame to include a wider choice: she could provide five boxes to tick rather than one, etc. Specific details of questionnaire design will be covered in Chapter 4.

CONSTRUCT VALIDITY

It is clear that there is considerable potential latitude in the design of a questionnaire to measure something such as the quality of a relationship. The actual type and numbers of individual items can vary considerably. How does the researcher know when they have got it right? How does one know that what one set out to measure is actually being measured, in this case the quality of a relationship? This is where construct validity comes to the rescue.

Failure to show any connection between asthma and parental relationships could be:

• because one does not exist (i.e. the hypothesis is wrong)
• because there has been a failure to measure adequately the quality of relationships (or asthma).

It is impossible to know which of the two is correct. However, if on the other hand, a correlation between asthma and quality of life *is* found then not only does this support the original hypothesis but it also indicates that the operationalization must have worked and is therefore in some sense valid. Of course, it may not have measured precisely what was intended but having shown a connection there is obviously some relationship there that can be pursued.

Let us take this argument through its steps again. Say there is a hypothesis that:

Wimps are only found among men.

1. First, a research design and a sample. Let us take the next consecutive 100 men and 100 women who consult, check who is a wimp and compare the two groups.
2. The variables, namely gender and wimpishness, need to be operationalized. Men and women can be identified from case records; only people over 18 will be eligible. It is a little-known yet long-established fact that cats abreact to wimps: a cat's reactions can therefore be used as an indicator of wimpishness. A cat's behaviour can be observed when these 200 people enter the consulting room.
3. The data is collected. Pickles, the surgery cat, ran out of the room when 7 out of the 100 men entered and when 2 of the 100 women entered.
4. Thus, looked at formally, either the initial hypothesis has been disproved (because it held that wimps were never found amongst women) or the cat has not proved to be a very valid instrument. Which is it? Let us try a new cat.
5. A new cat is hired and the experiment repeated. This cat runs out of the room when 6 of the men enter but never when a woman enters. The hypothesis is confirmed. And there can be some confidence that the new cat can somehow identify wimps better than the old one. (The cat may in fact be detecting the presence of aftershave—but whatever it does, it does better than the old cat.)

Now apply the same logic to Dr Warmhands' relationship questionnaire. Assume she uses her two-item questionnaire to assess quality of relationships. If she has allowed a two-point response set and scores these 0 or 1 then adding the two items together she gets a scale of 0 to 2 for quality of marriage. Let us assume the overall results are as follows:

20 asthmatic children: average marriage score   = 1.3
20 eczematous children: average marriage score = 1.4

The quality of relationships in her control group is slightly better, but hardly very much. She would be safe in saying there was no difference. What does this imply?

- either her hypothesis is mistaken
- or her relationship instrument was too crude to pick up the subtleties she was after.

Now consider some other results:

20 asthmatic children: average marriage score   = 0.3
20 eczematous children: average marriage score = 1.8

The results, and hence implications, are very different. She might still rightly be sceptical of her 'relationship' instrument, but it has certainly picked something up. She might wish to proceed to another study in which she can ask: What is it exactly about a relationship that has been identified? Is it something to do with rows specifically? Is it something to do with communication? She will need new hypotheses and new instruments to refine what she has discovered, but it does look as if, in this study, there really is an association between marital relations and childhood asthma.

In this way, a questionnaire is sufficient if it can help identify links between variables at both an empirical and theoretical level. The thought behind the hypothesis was that perhaps poor marital background actually caused or exacerbated asthma. Thus:

$$\text{poor parental interaction} \quad \rightarrow \quad \text{asthma}$$

These concepts were operationalized and measured. Thus:

$$\begin{array}{ccc}
\text{poor parental interaction} & & \text{asthma} \\
\Downarrow & & \Downarrow \\
\text{questionnaire} & \rightrightarrows & \text{peak flow}
\end{array}$$

A relationship was then found between the questionnaire findings and the peak flow reading. Assuming this has not occurred by chance—and this is established by statistical techniques explored in Chapter 9—an interesting finding has been uncovered because the link between the very specific measures indicates a link between the more fuzzy concepts. This phenomenon is called *construct validity* because it is known from the correlation between the measures that the hypothesis or construct has some validity.

The above examples are rather simple because they are based on only a two-variable relationship (parental relationships and asthma). In practice, construct validity is usually explored in the context of several supposedly related variables. Thus, for instance, it can be seen from the above example that if there is a positive correlation between the relationship questionnaire and asthma there is some support for the value of the relationship concept and how it was operationalized. But if, in addition, the questionnaire was used to identify couples with and without marital problems and then compared these for depression, and again a correlation was found, there is even more support for the concept and its operationalization. Clearly this process can go on and on, each new variable which can be linked to the initial concept reinforcing its validity, and gradually establishing a matrix of corroborative support for all the variables.

Construct validity is therefore important in two ways:

• When dealing with rather woolly concepts it offers some supportive evidence that the operationalization is adequate.
• Because research is ultimately about building hypotheses into wider explanatory models, construct validity provides the bridge between measuring

things and developing wider theories (often containing many variables) about the world.

If a positive correlation between two variables is found it is not the end of the research process but a sort of beginning. What has really been shown? What concept did the indicator really measure? Like a bloodhound following a scent, the researcher has to decide constantly in which direction to go. If a trail has no scent should it be abandoned or examined even more closely for a scent that may have been missed? If on the other hand a scent is discovered, its direction must be determined and then pursued.

Usually in research, data is collected on more than two variables so that if a trail is found it can be explored further without immediately going back to collect more data. Thus, if there does seem to be a correlation between parental relationships and asthma, the data can be used to ask additional questions:

Does it hold for boys and girls?

Is it age related?

And so on.

In this sense, research is never completed: it goes on, one question leading to another, one finding suggesting another or a new line of enquiry.

SUMMARY

This chapter has dealt with the process by which the abstract terms or concepts in a research design are transposed into practical measuring procedures. These stages are:

1. Operationalizing individual concepts to create measurable indicators.
2. Paying attention to the validity of this operationalization by checking wherever possible by:

• face validity
• convergent validity.

3. Checking to see if there is a correlation between elements in the hypothesis.

• if there is not a correlation:
    (a) discuss or change the hypothesis
    (b) rethink the operationalization
    (c) add some more checks for validity.
• if there is a correlation:
    (a) there is some construct validity
    (b) proceed to refine the hypothesis
    (c) refine and further develop the operationalization
    (d) use the new measures to collect data
    (e) check for new correlations.

SUGGESTED TASKS

1. Design and carry out a study to assess the reliability of sphygmomanometers both in the surgery and in doctors' bags. You might also try inter-person variability in the reading of a blood pressure.

2. For the next 10 investigations you order, try to predict the result. See if your clinical impression is as valid as the test.

ANSWERS TO EXERCISES

EXERCISE 3.1

Concept	Indicator
income	monthly net salary
elderly	aged over 65
women	presence of a vagina
	reported gender
stress	galvanic skin resistance
	heart rate
chronic illness	on disability register
	reports long-standing illness
GP workload	length of surgeries
	number of patients seen
referral rate	patients sent to out-patients
blood pressure	sphygmomanometer reading

EXERCISE 3.2

1. Aged over 65; any glycosuria?

2. (Difficult ... what is meant by concentration?) Each patient could be given a short message by a receptionist to give to the doctor. Doctor recalls message at end of consultation. Recall in first half-hour of surgery compared with last half-hour.

3. Compare the numbers over 65 in your age–sex register.

4. Identify high and low stressed patients by a stress questionnaire: compare their consultation rates from notes over last year. (Remember to balance your groups—high consulters are more likely to enter your sample if you use surgery patients.)

5. Divide hand movement into 'types', for example

• over chest, flat
• over chest, fisted
• not over chest.

For patients presenting with chest pain record type of hand movement, then make diagnosis, e.g. with ECG; does a particular hand movement correlate with ECG ischaemic changes? (If it does then there is some construct validity to the concept of 'diagnostic hand movements' which might be worth exploring further.)

EXERCISE 3.3

Question 1: Face validity.
Question 2: Convergent (concurrent) validity.
Question 3: Convergent (predictive) validity.
Question 4: Convergent (concurrent) validity.
Question 5: Face validity.

4 Collecting data

The last chapter dealt with deciding how you might go about measuring things. Having made those decisions you are almost ready to go 'into the field' to measure things in practice. But before you do so you have to give some thought to how you are going to collect your data. 'Data' are 'out there'. You will need some sort of 'net' to bring data in: the net must be the right size and its mesh dimensions appropriate for the data you want to capture. This chapter deals with designing this net for collecting data.

COLLECTING AND CLASSIFYING DATA

It is reported that if a blind person is given his or her sight back, initially they can only see a blur. Gradually they begin to recognize objects and eventually they can 'see'.

Sensory data surround us in an undiscriminated mass. As perceptual processes develop—usually in childhood—this blur of information begins to be organized and separate objects, colours, textures, sounds, and so on can be identified. In effect, being able to see is not simply allowing images to flood the retina—that would produce a haze—but using the brain to organize and select elements of visual data so that a recognizable picture can be identified. Of course there must be a sensory input through the retina, but the image is 'manufactured' in the visual cortex.

Research is exactly the same. Out there are data, masses and masses of the stuff. And one of the commonest mistakes of those not versed in research methods is to imagine that research is about having a data receptor—like a retina—that will enable giant spoonfuls of data to be captured.

'I've collected serum rhubarb estimations on over 600 patients.'
'Have you? I've done it on over 800!'
'Wow! What a big research grant/team/programme you must have!'

But so what? Chapter 1 stressed that you must start your research with a question. This is the point when perseverance pays off. Certainly you will need to collect data, but the research question (together with the research design, Chapter 2, and how the concepts were operationalized, Chapter 3) will help decide which data needs collecting and how it is going to be organized into a picture.

Data collection always involves some selectivity or organization; collecting 'random' data is feasible but clearly absurd. Nevertheless it is useful to distinguish between the collection of data and their categorization.

It would seem reasonable to plan to categorize data before their collection, so obtaining only the exact data that are required. However, in general practice research, especially when collecting data from people, there may be good grounds for actually collecting rather undifferentiated data and doing the sorting and categorization later, away from the heat of the moment.

Let us consider two examples of measuring how satisfied patients are with their last consultation in general practice.

1. Tape record a one hour interview with a patient in which you ask them to talk about their last consultation, its good points and bad points, and about their views of general practice in general. Let the patient do most of the talking: only prompt with open-ended questions or facilitative statements.

2. Give a patient a questionnaire to complete. The questionnaire contains the question:

> 'Were you satisfied with your last consultation?'   yes ❑   no ❑
>
>   (Please tick the appropriate box)

With both of these approaches the data are 'out there' mixed in with all sorts of other data, such as opinions on baked beans, politicians, and shrubs. The research question boils down to abstracting from this amorphous mass whether or not the patient was satisfied with the last consultation.

In example 1, the data collected in an hour-long tape recording were sufficiently focused so as to be mainly about general practice, but it was not sufficiently categorized to answer the research question (Was the patient satisied?) without further work by the researcher to disentangle relevant data from background 'noise'.   In example 2, on the other hand, the data were collected and categorized at exactly the same time. Indeed, by giving the patient a self-administered questionnaire the patients themselves did the organizing of data (into categories chosen by the researcher).

The fact that questionnaires that are self-administered and 'structured' (in that they require the patient simply to answer closed questions) are a popular way of collecting data is no doubt primarily due to the ease by which data collection and organization are done in one simple exercise (using the respondent as a sort of unpaid research assistant). However, this sort of data collection and organization has limitations and, in many ways, example 1 may give a 'better' result. Example 2 depends on the patient as untrained researcher to do the classification. But is this wise? Patients may misinterpret the question, they might think the question is about whether they got well or were given a prescription or whatever, and answer accordingly. Example 1 allows the data to be classified according to consistent and more rigorous criteria. Moreover it allows the asking of potentially more interesting questions such as 'What was it exactly that the patient found satisfying?'

The choice is therefore between relatively complex data collection methods which may produce good quality data, but where complexity means sample size may be restricted, and simpler techniques which allow large numbers of cases to make up for any insensitivity in the measuring instrument. Whichever method is used will be strongly influenced by the precise nature of the research question being asked. Without doubt, collecting data on patients' ages is best done using a question that asks the patient to give an answer properly categorized into the exact number of years; on the other hand, the validity of a response to the question 'What is the quality of your life?' that involved ticking one of two boxes is likely to be limited: these latter sorts of data are better collected in a more un-differentiated form.

In this chapter the concern is with data collection, but inevitably some methods of collection involve quite elaborate pre-classification, as explained above, whereas others tend to deal with fairly raw material. The subsequent steps of completing categorization and carrying out further manipulation will be pursued in Chapter 6.

TYPES OF DATA COLLECTION

A new weight-reducing drug called Skinnyfax has recently been brought on to the market. Results from trials indicate that it might be beneficial, although it is still unclear how it works. Does it actually cause weight reduction in everyone? Does it produce weight reduction by appetite suppression or increasing basic metabolic rate? And what are its side-effects? There have been some reports of raised blood pressure. Dr Adrian Slim decides to set up a small research study evaluating its impact in the context of general practice.

His sample consists of patients who consult with him whose weight is above the 90th percentile for their age. The design involves the patients being random-ized between an experimental group which receives the drug, and a group which acts as a control. (The patients will be asked if they agree to this procedure.) Part of the study will involve collecting baseline information on a range of topics so as to identify the level and nature of change (if any) produced by the drug. Dr Slim will need to collect information on patients' eating habits, weight, blood pressure, side-effects, and so on, and record any changes in the experimental and control groups.

What methods are there for collecting the necessary data? Figure 4.1 shows the possibilities.

Each method involves collecting data at different levels of prior categor-ization: data collected by relatively unstructured means will require later struc-turing, while data collected by structured means will be virtually ready for analysis.

Let us see how these different methods might work for the data needed for the Skinnyfax study, especially the data on eating habits.

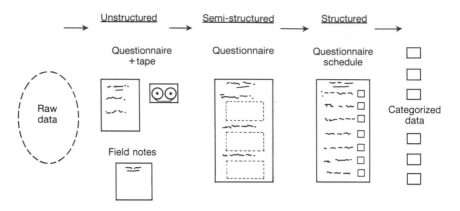

Fig. 4.1 Data collection methods.

UNSTRUCTURED TECHNIQUES

These divide into observation and interview.

Observation

When social anthropologists study a community they often use techniques of unstructured observation. They do not want to intrude into what is going on, such as by asking questions, because these might cause someone to change their behaviour; the preferred technique is therefore observation. Second, they want their observations to be unstructured because if they were to structure their collection of data using a classification system devised before they arrived in the community they might miss something important. Thus, they start with a blank piece of paper headed 'field notes' and write down the things they see. To stay within the bounds of the possible, some structuring is of course necessary, and so the researchers will only write down what they believe might be significant in the context of their interests. Arguably, this low-level selection of what to record is better and more sensitive than having a list of pre-set questions that need answering.

In similar fashion, when finding out what people eat, there are clear advantages in making an actual observation of what they really do eat. Thus, like an anthropologist, Dr Slim could visit their homes and, without preconceptions of what he might find, observe their behaviour. In practice this would no doubt be impractical but the basis of this sort of data collection, if it were feasible, is worth spelling out. (While this procedure may be unsuitable for this particular study topic it may be useful elsewhere—such as in the consulting room.)

If Dr Slim were accepted as a fly on the wall he would presumably get a better idea of eating habits—perhaps the husband or father gets twice as much as anyone else—whereas a questionnaire may simply elicit some general gloss such as 'we all eat the same'. Equally, going in without preconceptions such as a structured list of questions will enable surprising or unexpected events to be recorded.

After he has made his observations there are three things he can do with them:

1. Use these accounts as descriptive studies in their own right which offer insights into the phenomena under study, and write them up as such (i.e. as purely qualitative descriptive accounts).
2. Read them through carefully and use the insights they afford as the basis for a more traditional structured questionnaire to be used on a larger sample.
3. Analyse the field notes and transpose 'qualitative' data into quantitative by techniques described in Chapter 6.

Interview

What happens if the phenomena Dr Slim wishes to explore are not behaviours but mental processes such as attitudes, beliefs, or values? The method of data collection chosen is exactly analogous to unstructured observation, only this time, instead of using field notes to record data, he would use a tape-recorder. With observational techniques he could observe a meal; with interview techniques he obviously cannot rely on the patient suddenly talking about their attitude to food when the tape recorder is placed in front of them. Instead he would have to create the necessary conditions which encourage and enable them to talk about eating: this is done by a series of open-ended questions, prompts, and facilitating responses, which written down beforehand would constitute an *unstructured questionnaire*. It might look something like this:

Eating habits questionnaire
Respondent's name:
Date:
Time:
Tape number:

Tell me about your food shopping?
Who does it? Always? Where? How often?
Do you decide in advance what to buy?
What sorts of things do you buy?
Always? For special occasions?   etc.

Dr Slim may not need to use many of these questions, should a respondent cover the topics spontaneously for him. Or if the respondent starts to talk about the role of money in determining shopping patterns it might be inappropriate to return to the planned topics, so instead the new lead would be pursued. In effect the questionnaire is just a series of prompts to ensure that the interview does not dry up, otherwise it is allowed to take its own course.

Again the results of the interview on the tape can be used as the basis of a descriptive account, transformed into quantitative data, or used to create a structured questionnaire.

SEMI-STRUCTURED TECHNIQUES

These, as their name implies, fall midway between unstructured and structured techniques. The most important is the *semi-structured questionnaire* in which the questions are fairly well structured but unstructured responses are allowed. In other words all respondents will get the same questions but as they will be open-ended everyone will provide answers different in both content and form. Thus the question, 'Where do you do your shopping?', might elicit the response 'Sainsburys' from one person but a five-minute monologue on grocery retailing from another. The results of semi-structured questionnaires can be analysed in the same way as unstructured.

STRUCTURED TECHNIQUES

Structured techniques collect data which is pre-categorized, with perhaps the best known being the structured questionnaire, but many forms of data collection fall into this mode. Indeed any piece of paper on which is written pre-categorized data is a structured technique. These are known as *schedules*.

Let us consider different forms of schedule.

A clinical schedule

The Skinnyfax study requires Dr Slim to collect some clinical data. These might include information on the patient's weight, height, blood pressure, and perhaps some laboratory investigations. He decides to collect most of these during the consultation. To record the data he will need to design a schedule. How might this look?

It would probably be on a single sheet of paper. It would require a title, if only to distinguish it from other schedules lying around the surgery . The first entry would probably be the patient's name, together with a code number which the researcher would devise. The value of having a code number as an identifier should become clearer later, but briefly, the data are more than likely to be computerized and computers are not very good at handling people's names; instead a three-digit number would easily enable the identification of up to 999 individual patients. Dr Slim might want the date on which he did the examination, and of course places to record the clinical data. The finished product might look something like this:

Skinnyfax study: baseline clinical data
Patient's name: Code number:

Date:

Height (metres):
Weight (kilograms):

Blood pressure:

Haemoglobin:
Serum cholesterol:

(Presumably laboratory findings can be added later when the results are returned.)

The advantage of having such a schedule is that nothing is forgotten in the data collection and data are not spread over odd bits and pieces of paper. In addition, if the schedule is carefully designed the data in the boxes can be used directly to create a data file on a computer: the value of this will become apparent in a later chapter where coding of a questionnaire is described.

The clinical schedule can be expanded to include data collected in the evaluation phase. Indeed the schedule could be so designed as to bring all the data on each case together on the same record.

An extraction schedule

It may be possible to obtain study data from other written sources, especially case notes. Again the source is likely to include far too much data so some sort of schedule must be designed—in this case what is called an extraction schedule—so as to obtain the desired data. Its form is likely to be the same as the clinical schedule outlined above. Indeed, if the case notes were to contain the relevant data exactly the same schedule could be used.

Case notes are the most likely source of written data. But as case notes are primarily used for clinical and administrative purposes, the information recorded will be structured by these aims. For example, the breadth of information for a research investigation on eating habits is unlikely to be available unless some careful attempt has been made to record such data in the past. However, the case notes could be used in this study for validity checks for weight and for other clinical information such as blood pressure.

A structured questionnaire

Often the data to be collected has to be obtained not from patients' bodies nor from written records but from what exists in the patient's mind (attitudes, moods, values, beliefs, ...). The common technique for doing this is the structured or standardized questionnaire where the range of questions is structured, meaning that choice of answers is restricted. This approach stands in contrast to the unstructured interview where there is no set order and no schedule, and the researcher is not necessarily looking for exactly the same information from each respondent.

Questionnaires are exactly analogous to any other schedule but, because it is people who are being interrogated, they must be more carefully set out and worded. Thus the question 'Height:' which was sufficient on the clinical schedule would have to be reworded: perhaps 'What is your height in metres?'. In addition, care must be taken in the design of the questionnaire to ensure maximum response rates. The sphygmomanometer is not usually in the habit of saying 'I don't think I want to measure this particular blood pressure', whereas people do have an unfortunate disposition to say no to the best-intentioned research studies.

The use of a standardized questionnaire is most appropriate for collecting information:

- from a large number of people
- from a relatively homogeneous group of people who tend to share the same general perspective and characteristics
- in situations where you already know enough about the subject and the kinds of respondents so that you know what to ask and how to ask it.

The major limitation of this approach is when it is used with groups of respondents who do not necessarily share your values and views, and thus the assumptions that are incorporated into the questionnaire are invalid. For example, if you are looking at patterns of eating habits and the factors that influence them, you might assume that people's concern about matters of health are of paramount importance. However, this might be an invalid assumption and only reflect your concerns as a professional rather than the values and priorities of your respondents.

The questions in the structured schedule can be given to the respondents in at least two ways. The questionnaire can be given directly to the respondent for them to complete themselves (*a self-administered questionnaire*) or it can be given by a trained intermediary (*an interviewer-administered questionnaire*). Self-administered questionnaires are particularly useful for collecting relatively straightforward information from a large sample, quickly and cheaply. On the other hand an interviewer-administered questionnaire tends to produce a higher response rate (80 per cent on average) and better-quality information. Also, the questionnaire itself could be more complicated as the interviewer would be on hand to explain the questions. However, it is more time-consuming and expensive, not least because you have to recruit, pay, and train the interviewers.

QUESTION 4.1

Dr Slim feels that his survey on eating habits should be simple and he is confident that the use of a standardized questionnaire is appropriate. However, he has to decide on how to gather the information. Should he use:

* a self-administered postal questionnaire?
* an interviewer-administered questionnaire?

Self-administered questionnaires can be handed out to patients in person, in the surgery, but this restricts the sample to patients who consult; alternatively they can be sent by post. Certainly postal questionnaires have some advantages over interviews:

* they are generally cheaper and quicker
* they are useful with a large and widely distributed sample, such as a national sample.

However, there are also some disadvantages with a postal questionnaire:

* the response is rarely as high as interview studies as there is less incentive to respond— the average response rate in a postal questionnaire is around 50–60 per cent.
* the quality of response to the questionnaire may be variable and there is no guarantee that the selected individual will be the member of the household who has filled it in.

If a postal questionnaire is used, emphasis would be placed on trying to maximize the response rate. Much will depend on the covering letter that is sent with the questionnaire and in addition follow-up reminders will need to be sent out.

For example, here is a letter which might be sent with a postal questionnaire on health habits:

Dear Sir or Madam,

We are writing to ask for your help with a health survey which the Rundown Health Authority is carrying out with Smallbrick University.

It is the responsibility of the Health Authority to promote health and prevent disease as well as to treat illness when it occurs. We want to find out more about the general health of our community and about factors that may affect people's health such as smoking, diet, exercise, and drinking. By filling in this questionnaire about your health you will help us to do this and, in due course, to improve the health of the community.

We obviously cannot send out questionnaires to every person living in Rundown so we have carefully selected a random sample which should be representative of the district as a whole. It is important to us that you fill in your questionnaire and return it as your replies are essential in building up the overall picture.

You will find that most questions are simple to answer, requiring just a tick in a box, although any extra comments you may wish to make will be welcomed.

Your reply will be handled in strict confidence. This means that your name will not appear on the questionnaire, it will be handled only by authorized members of the research staff, and your answers will not be seen by your GP or any other person. The questionnaire will be shredded after use and no individuals will be identified or identifiable in any reports or publications. When you have returned the questionnaire there will be no further communication from us.

The replies will be analysed in the Health Services Research Unit of Smallbrick University and we will be grateful if you return your completed questionnaire in the enclosed envelope.

May we thank you in advance for the time and trouble taken in completing this questionnaire.

Yours faithfully,

The letter tells the respondent:

- who is carrying out the survey
- why the survey is being carried out and its value
- why the individual has been selected
- how to fill in the questionnaire
- about confidentiality and anonymity
- where to return the questionnaire.

On most occasions one attempted contact with the respondent is not sufficient to obtain a good enough response rate in a postal survey. The first follow-up, usually a short letter or a postcard, is sent two to three weeks after the first letter and questionnaire. The main aim is to jog the memory of those who intended to complete the questionnaire but have either forgotten or have not found the time.

The second follow-up (if one is used—by now diminishing returns are likely to have set in) usually involves a more persuasive covering letter with another copy of the questionnaire. It too has the aim of reminding respondents, although it is also aimed at the hard core of non-responders, attempting to persuade them to take part. Using more than two follow-ups is not usually cost-effective, in that the time and money spent on sending out letters and paying for return envelopes does not justify the small increase in the response rate.

In general the following factors are believed to increase response rates (and conversely their absence to decrease them):

- the more independent and prestigious the sponsoring body (universities tend to do better than commercial market research organizations)
- the brevity of the questionnaire (the shorter the better)
- identification of the respondent with the area of the research (a questionnaire on skin diseases will elicit a better response from those concerned about their skin than those not)
- ease of completion (clear instructions, easy and rapid marking, a stamped addressed return envelope)
- payment or financial incentive (though these are rare).

After weighing up his choices Dr Slim decides to use a postal questionnaire to assess his patients' eating habits.

HOW DO YOU CONSTRUCT A QUESTIONNAIRE?

A self-administered questionnaire needs careful thought as you will not be able to depend on the skills of the interviewer to mediate between the questionnaire and the respondent when the data are collected. How do you go about it? There are several important elements to be considered.

A title

The questionnaire should have a title not only to identify it for your benefit, but also so that the respondent will have some idea of what it is about. Keep it short and clear: 'Satisfaction survey'or 'Self-medication questionnaire', for example. Dr Slim chooses 'Eating patterns questionnaire'.

An address

If you are carrying out a postal survey you should provide an address somewhere in the questionnaire, often just under the title. Do not rely on the address on a covering letter as these get mislaid. Even for questionnaires handed out in the surgery it is useful to have a name and/or address in case the patient inadvertently walks out without handing it in. Dr Slim puts, under his title:

please return to:
Dr Adrian Slim
Puddledown Health Centre

An identifier

There should be a box somewhere near the beginning of the questionnaire in which can be written the respondent's code number. This is used as an identifier so that one respondent's questionnaire can easily be distinguished from any other. This is particularly useful in postal surveys for sending out reminder letters or postcards (to those not replying to a first mailing), or in constructing the data file (see Chapter 6). Dr Slim's survey is of 500 patients so he places a box to take a three-digit number in the top right-hand corner of the questionnaire where it is easily visible.

Some instructions

The first section of any questionnaire should also tell respondents something about the survey and how to complete the questionnaire. This should be as clear and as simple as possible. Dr Slim prefaces the questions with the following remarks:

> We are carrying out a survey of people's eating habits in this practice and we would be grateful for your help. Can you please answer the following questions. Most simply require a tick in the appropriate boxes.
>
> All your answers will be treated in the strictest confidence. Thank you for helping.

Alternatively, in a postal questionnaire some of these details could be described in the covering letter.

The questions

The next stage involves constructing the actual questions. This requires the identification of the particular topics needed for the questionnaire, and then these need formalizing into specific questions.

Topics

Dr Slim decides that he wants to divide the topic area of study into the food that is bought, the way food is prepared for meals and the type of meals that are eaten. He is also interested in social and demographic characteristics of his patients and how they vary with eating habits; so he adds social class, income, age, sex, household size, and marital status to his checklist.

Specific questions

The specific questions asked will be related to the topics and items listed previously. There are some general rules for asking questions:

- keep the questions as short and as specific as possible
- use simple language
- avoid leading questions
- avoid inviting a single response to what are in fact two questions: 'Do you like meat and vegetables?'

Many questions are straightforward, especially ones that elicit simple facts. For example, 'How old are you?' is clear and unambiguous. If the questionnaire consists of these types of questions then it is only necessary to make sure the wording is clear, the question is answerable, an appropriate place or box is indicated for the response, and all questions are neatly laid out.

QUESTION 4.2

Which of the following questions could be used in your survey?
1. Do you have milk delivered or do you drive to the supermarket?
2. Is the meat/fish you buy usually: fresh salmon, caviar, veal, or pheasant?

3. Please list all the restaurants/cafes you have eaten in, what you ate, who you were with, and how much you spent?
4. Should working people have a regular, balanced diet?
5. What are your shops like?
6. Do you prefer high levels of saturated or polyunsaturated fatty acids in your diet?
7. Why do you think being overweight is unhealthy?
8. You don't think doctors should give more advice on smoking, do you?

None of these questions is suitable—there are problems with all of them.
1. is a double question that contains two different parts
2. offers a restricted and limited choice that may be irrelevant to the group being investigated
3. contains too many different questions—they need to be separated
4. contains too many words whose meaning is unclear, such as 'working', 'regular', and 'balance'
5. is too broad and needs to be more specific
6. has too much jargon
7. is a leading question
8. the researcher's preferences and biases influence the answer.

Questions often seek opinions, and these tend to require a little more thought. A knowledge of the different types of questions and some possible formats can help in designing these sorts of questions.

Questions divide into two broad types, *closed* and *open*. The former, fixed choice, or what are sometimes called *pre-coded*, questions require the respondent to place his or her answer within a given range of choices. The latter are 'open' to any answer the respondent wishes to give.

Closed questions

To a certain extent the exact choice of question format will depend on the nature of the study in hand, although much of the choice is fairly arbitrary. Try different sorts. Here are some formats you might want to consider:

Question 1. Do you think your diet can influence your health? (Please tick.)

yes ❑

no ❑

The yes/no response is perhaps the most basic question format that can be used. As long as the subject is appropriate it is fairly easy and quick to answer. The only problem comes, as in all closed questions, when there is not a response category to fit the respondent's view. A not uncommon reaction when answering yes/no questions is to feel unsure (Can diet really influence health...?). With only two choices the uncertain respondent is either forced into ticking the box which is nearest their view, or ignoring the question. The choice for the researcher is therefore between forcing a decision (perhaps with a statement in the introduction requesting respondents to tick the box which is nearest their view), or providing a third box for the undecided. Thus:

Question 2.   Do you think your diet can influence your health? (Please tick.)

yes   ❏

no   ❏

uncertain   ❏

A problem with the above question is that there is no way of differentiating between those who think diet is very influential and those who think it has a minor role, as both will have ticked 'yes'. A common way round this is to offer a *scale*: perhaps, 'yes, a lot' and 'yes, a little'. Here is another example:

Question 3.   Are you eating a different diet from last year?
(Please circle answer)

Definitely	1
Small change only	2
No change	3
Not sure	4.

Here the respondent is offered a scale consisting of three numbers to record the extent of the change (plus a number for the unsure). This question could just as easily have been answered by ticking boxes; the advantage of using numbers is that these digits can be transferred directly to the data file when the questionnaires are being processed (see Chapter 6). The disadvantage with numbers is that it might appear confusing to the respondent that 'unsure' (a 4) is somehow 'more' than 'no change' (a 3).

Another common question format is that based around what is called a Likert scale:

Question 4.   To what extent do you agree with the following statement: 'Fat people tend to be happier than thin people.'

Strongly agree	1
Agree	2
Uncertain	3
Disagree	4
Strongly disagree	5.

Usually the scale consists of a number of statements (or items) which are both positive (in this case favouring obesity) and negative. Scores are allocated to each response on each item and so long as each question refers to the same phenomenon, in this case obesity, the scores can be summed (after allowing for whether the question was in a negative or positive format).

Another variant of a self-administered scale is the *visual analogue scale* where respondents are asked to mark a point (by a cross or a circle) on a scale to indicate their answer.

Question 5. Do you think that obesity is important in causing ill-health? Please mark a point on the line below.

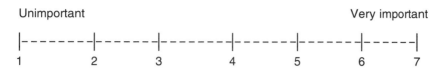

Unimportant   Very important

|-------+------+------+------+------+-----|
1   2   3   4   5   6   7

Another type of graphic rating scale is the semantic differential. This is another way of identifying respondents' attitudes to particular concepts. For example, if the concept being explored was obesity, the scale might look like this:

Question 6. How do you think of obese people? Look at the pair of words given below and mark on the line, between each pair, the point that represents your view.
For example, if you have to consider whether obese people tend to be funny or serious, and your view is that they are somewhere in the middle but perhaps a bit on the serious side you might answer as below:

Funny | – – – – – – – – – – – × – – – – – | Serious

Now please do the same for the following pairs of adjectives.

Good | – – – – – – – – – – – – – – – – | Bad
Attractive | – – – – – – – – – – – – – – – | Ugly
Healthy | – – – – – – – – – – – – – – – | Unhealthy
Happy | – – – – – – – – – – – – – – – – | Unhappy
Relaxed | – – – – – – – – – – – – – – – | Anxious

The example shows that the semantic differential consists of pairs of adjectives which are opposites. Each respondent is asked to mark on the scales their rating of obesity in relation to the adjectives involved. The position can then be given scores of 1 to 5. Each scale can be treated independently, or they are often combined to see if a more general factor can be identified.

Another strategy is to ask respondents to grade or order items:

Question 7. Which of the following vegetables do you prefer to eat?
(Please rank in order of preference)

Potatoes   Carrots   Peas   Beans   Cabbage

1st choice   – – – – – – – – – – – – – – – – –
2nd choice   – – – – – – – – – – – – – – – – –
3rd choice   – – – – – – – – – – – – – – – – –

This sort of question is useful in determining respondent's priorities though choosing more than three or four items from a long list can be a difficult task.

Yet another type of question involves dividing the respondents into groups and directing one group to another question:

Question 8.   Do you eat meat?   yes ❏
                                             no ❏
            If 'yes', 'Do you eat meat every day?   yes ❏
                                                               no ❏
            If 'no', 'Have you ever eaten meat?   yes ❏
                                                        no, never ❏

This is an example of a filter question where the respondents are divided into sub-groups and asked different clusters of questions. The question could then divide into other sub-groups such as by type of meat eaten, although it is better in a self-administered questionnaire to ensure that the questioning is not too complicated.

Questions may also be included in the questionnaire to check the consistency or *internal reliability* of the questionnaire. For example, this question:

Question 9. Government regulation of additives in food is desirable.

                        (Please circle answer)
            Agree   1
            Disagree   2
            Don't know   3

might be followed later in the questionnaire by:

Question 10. Additives in food should not be regulated by the government.   (Please circle answer)
            Agree   1
            Disagree   2
            Don't know   3

Such questions act as checks on the performance of the respondent. If the above questions elicited contradictory responses it might suggest that the respondent is guessing (perhaps because the question is not understood) or is not taking the exercise seriously. Either of these would be a signal to treat the respondent as a 'non-responder'.

Open questions

Open questions do not constrain the respondent to answer according to the limited response set of the closed question.

Question 11. Do you think that the diet you eat can influence your health?

            _

            _

This is the same as Question 1, above, but because a fixed-choice response is not provided the respondent is invited to answer in any way he or she likes. The main advantage of such open-ended questions is that they do not make prior judgements about the way the respondent should answer. The main disadvantage is that they are difficult and time-consuming to code and analyse. In many ways they are probably better suited to an interview survey rather than a self-administered questionnaire, in that the interviewer will have the opportunity of further exploring partial or unclear answers.

The ending

Sometimes, especially with lots of closed questions, respondents can get angry or frustrated that the available questions or limited choice of responses do not cover their particular interest or view. It is therefore often useful to offer a very open question right at the end:

Question 12. Do you have any further points to make about this topic?

— —

Many respondents will ignore this question, others will let off steam, and yet others will offer insightful comments on the subject of the research or the details of the questionnaire. Thus, while the responses are often of limited value in so far as the specifics of the questionnaire are concerned, they can be therapeutic for both respondent and researcher.

Respondents usually fill in questionnaires for no personal benefit: they are doing the researcher a favour and it is appropriate to thank them at the end:

Thank you for helping with this study.

The layout

Having designed all the components of the questionnaire, the next stage is to put them all together. It seems hardly necessary to say that the questionnaire should appear neat, clear, and attractive. There is often a compromise to be made between spacing it out well and not letting it appear too long. In addition, some of the items will need to be ordered.

QUESTION 4.3

In what order do you place the following questions?

1. What is your income?
2. Where do you buy your shopping?   local shops
                                            supermarket
3. What are the best ways of staying healthy?

4. How do you get to the shops?   car

                                          bus

                                          other.

The usual order is to place the more impersonal and easy to answer questions at the start to enlist co-operation and gain interest; in this case that is Question 2. This is usually followed by questions such as 4 that are less interesting. The 'sensitive' 1 and the open-ended 3 are usually left to the end of the study. There is also a need to see the questionnaire as a whole, so linking phrases are necessary to ensure a smooth link-up between sections. For example, the interviewer or the text might say:

The last question asked about the food you buy, the next group of questions looks at how you prepare and eat it.

Testing

The final stage of any questionnaire design is testing it for problems. It is vital that the whole research procedure is critically reviewed in the form of a *pilot* study; this is covered in the next chapter. But even before this testing it is important to examine critically the questionnaire which has been designed. The most experienced researcher is still fully capable of putting silly or unanswerable questions into a questionnaire and these can only be picked up by asking other people to check it over.

Ask your spouse, your partners, your receptionists to look over it, and, if it might apply to them, to try answering it. Listen carefully to their feedback and comments on how it was to be a respondent. Then try it on some patients (though not those who might get it in the study proper, as this might bias the result) and get their comments. Only when all say that it is clear and easy to answer are you in a position to go on to the pilot stage of the research.

A note on established instruments

It is not always necessary to devise your own questionnaire. A number of pre-packaged instruments already exist for measuring such common concepts as depression, quality of life, personality, health status, stress, intelligence, and so on, These questionnaires have been constructed using the same principles described above. Moreover, they have often been 'validated' by other researchers. These off-the-shelf questionnaires are extremely useful and you should be encouraged to try some of them, particularly for fairly well-defined phenomena such as depression that you are unlikely to operationalize in a significantly different way. Their main problem lies in their claimed validity: check to see whether they have been 'validated' on a population similar to the one that you intend to use them on—but bear in mind that your personally devised one-off questionnaire may have even less apparent validity.

SUMMARY

This chapter has principally dealt with the process of how to devise an instrument for collecting information. The stages involved with this data collection process are:
- consideration of qualitative as opposed to quantitative methods
- consideration of costs and benefits between choosing a self-administered and an interview survey
- designing a questionnaire.

SUGGESTED TASKS

1. Design a questionnaire to measure patient satisfaction with your repeat prescription system.
2. Design a schedule for evaluating and comparing the workload between partners.
3. Design a questionnaire which would identify difficulties your receptionists find with their work.

5 In the field

Previous chapters have described the basic principles of setting up a research project. Of course, in practice it is rarely as clear and logical—all sorts of things can, and do, go wrong. This chapter tries to give some ideas about the practical difficulties that can arise while you are 'out there' collecting data or trying to get the whole project under way. That said, the best way of learning about problems like this is actually to meet them when doing your own research: there is no substitute for getting hands-on experience.

THE PILOT STUDY

A research study very rarely runs entirely smoothly; there are always unexpected problems and difficulties. The solution is to try as far as possible to anticipate, minimize, or avoid these problems, and probably the most important way of doing this is to carry out a pilot study.

The pilot study is the dress rehearsal for the main study in which any fine tuning to the practical procedures takes place. It should therefore follow as closely as possible the design of the main study, except, of course, that it is carried out on a much smaller scale. The sample used should consist of people whose characteristics bear as much resemblance as possible to those that will be used in the main sample, though to prevent contamination no-one should be used who might be included in the main study's sample. Thereafter, the data collection procedures are run through as if this was the real thing.

In an apparently straightforward study it is tempting to skimp on or ignore the pilot. This is unwise. The best laid plans can have flaws: you will discover that some of the questionnaire is unintelligible, the receptionists did not know they should ask everyone a certain question, the case numbering system did not work, your partner forgot to collect the data, you lost the random number tables, and so on. The pilot is the evidence that the practical part of the data collection will actually work.

PLANNING AND PREPARATION

Preparation for the process of data collection involves not only designing an appropriate instrument for measurement but also considering and deciding upon the timetable for the data collection, and finding and recruiting any necessary staff.

Timetabling is important in any project. Draw up a schedule at the beginning so you can keep a check on progress. Very roughly, allow about one third of the time for planning, one third for data collection, and one third for analysis and writing up. In data collection you will need to allow for piloting and any printing necessary for the final questionnaire. Then you have to decide when to carry out the data collection and for how long.

QUESTION 5.1

You want to carry out a trial of Skinnyfax with your overweight patients over four consecutive weeks. Rank the following months in terms of suitability for the project:

- February
- August
- December
- October.

There is probably no ideal time. Eventually a compromise has to be reached between many factors such as:

- maximizing the likelihood of collecting the data required
- ensuring that there is a strong likelihood of collecting a truly representative sample of the population being studied.

February tends to be a busy month in most practices and the staff would not have the time to organize and run the trial then.

August would appear to be a generally quiet time—so quiet that in many practices patients and doctors go on holiday. Practices located in popular holiday areas may find that the opposite applies, and it may be the busiest time of the year with a flood of temporary residents. Whichever the local situation, there may be doubts as to the representativeness of the sample, as well as practical difficulties associated with the collection of the data.

December is a month which tends to be reasonably busy and partners tend not to be on holiday. Unfortunately, it might not be as convenient for patients who may not have the time near Christmas to fill in a questionnaire.

It would seem that October would be a more suitable month for the project without too many disruptions from holidays and without too much disturbances to the daily functioning of the practice. However, as pointed out, there is no ideal time. It depends on the type of project, the type of practice, the availability of help, limitations imposed by funding bodies, and so on. One can only aim for the best all-round compromise. Similarly, when thinking about the duration of the study there are many factors to consider.

QUESTION 5.2

You work in a small practice and recognize that to find a sample of 300 patients (including controls) within the specified time period you will need to recruit a number of other GPs. It appears that GPs see on average one obese person every two days. How many GPs will you need to recruit to your study?

1   5   10   20   100

One of the major constraints on the design of any project, especially if it involves the help of other people (as it usually does), such as patients, partners, colleagues, or staff, will be the limit to their enthusiasm, and hence their diligence in collecting the data. On the figures you have obtained, it looks as if something like 10 overweight patients will be identified by each GP every month. Thus, in addition to yourself and your partner you would need to recruit 28 GPs to do it in four weeks. Alternatively, you could extend the time period to two months and reduce the number of GPs to be recruited. Again, the compromise will be between recruiting large numbers of GPs to collect the data and facing the organizational problems that may be associated with collecting data from large numbers (allowing for follow-up, etc.), and recruiting a small number and expecting diligent data collection from them over what may be a long time period. You may decide that ten GPs collecting data over a three-month period appears to be a suitable compromise. However, if you find that you cannot recruit that many GPs, you may need to rethink the design of the study, especially the sizes of the samples, rather than extend the period of data collection from those GPs whose enthusiasm for the project will have finite limits.

Sufficient time must also be allowed for setting up the project, for last-minute administrative hitches, and for mounting the pilot study to try out the method.

Another practical problem that may occur, depending on the size of the project, is that of recruiting staff and training them. For the majority of projects mounted within primary care by GPs, especially those within their own practice, this will probably not be a problem. The staff used in the data collection will often be the practice staff such as receptionists, practice managers, and secretaries, adding yet another task to their many duties. Even so, they will still need careful explanations of what is expected of them, together with the rehearsal afforded by the pilot study.

THE PROJECT

Over coffee one day Dr Don Doolittle's attention is drawn to the fact that the female doctor in his partnership always finishes her surgery after the other partners.

He therefore decides to organize and design a project to see if female GPs have longer consultations with their patients than do male GPs.

TIME ANALYSIS FORM			
Date:		Name of GP:	
Time patient entered	Sex	Age	Time patient left

Fig. 5.1 Time analysis form.

He asks members of the local Young Practitioners Group to help, but before starting he decides to run a pilot study in his own practice.

He designs the form shown in Fig. 5.1, in which he hopes to record the length of all consultations over the course of a week.

QUESTION 5.3

How should he collect the information?

- get his receptionist to do it
- complete it himself at the end of each consultation
- hire a clerical research helper to sit outside his room.

The second option is probably preferable. The form is fairly simple, the information should be readily available: it just requires him to remember to do it.

TIME ANALYSIS FORM			
Date:		Name of GP:	
Time patient entered	Sex	Age	Time patient left
9.03	F	30 ish	9.12
9.12	F	7	9.15
9.15	M	10	–
–	M	10	–
–	F	25	–
–	–	–	–
–	M	–	–
10.45	M	50	10.53
			Surgery ended

Fig. 5.2 Time analysis form (completed).

Hiring research staff to help on a fairly simple study is just not worth the time, resources, and effort, especially if it can be carried out within the practice; besides, if Dr Doolittle does it he can keep a close eye on everything that happens.

In this instance Dr Doolittle decides to choose the first option, since he felt that this was a fairly simple task that his receptionist could easily fit in with her other duties. He then gets the sheet shown in Fig. 5.2 back from the receptionist.

She points out that the start of the next consultation may not be the same as the end of the previous one, since occasionally Dr Doolittle has odd gaps in his appointments, or makes a telephone call, and that sometimes patients can slip out without being seen. She also says that she was too busy between 9.25 and 10.20 on that Monday morning and that she had not had time to fill in those appointments, but, still, she does not think it will matter too much as she was sure she could remember most of them anyway.

QUESTION 5.4

Should Dr Doolittle:

- decide to choose an alternative method?
- carry on regardless since at least some of the times must be nearly right?
- sack the receptionist?

Hopefully he should ignore the last two options. He therefore decides to go back and choose the first method and fill in the form himself during surgery.

He completes the first two or three satisfactorily, but then realizes half way through the third surgery that he has forgotten to record any patients.

QUESTION 5.5

Should Dr Doolittle:

1. Try and estimate the start and finish times for the 10 patients he has seen so far?
2. Divide the time elapsed since surgery started by the number of patients seen to arrive at an average figure, and use this?
3. Forget about it for this surgery and hope to remember at the next?
4. Give himself a mental mark of 0 out of 10 for effort, and start all over again.

If he selected option 1, then probably he needs to reread the book so far.

Option 2 may not be as sloppy as it sounds. The problem would be that he does not know, at this stage, what sort of analysis will be used, and whether an 'average' time is suitable—it probably is not. Also he may not allow for time not consulting, such as telephone calls or time spent between consultations. All in all probably best avoided.

Option 3 is perfectly safe, but will he do any better next time? Is there not some way of ensuring that he remembers to start filling in the form at the start of the surgery—a note on his desk, a knot in his practice manager? Perhaps he can draw some lessons about the commitment that he is expecting from people, such as receptionists or other GPs, who have not even had the incentive of being directly involved in the planning of the project.

PROJECT NO. 2

Six months later, having completed his first project, Dr Doolittle decides to try and answer a more ambitious question:

Would reducing the number of patients seen in surgery improve the quality of the service offered?

He decides to take a sample of GPs in Fundless Health District. He sends the following letter to all 123 GPs on the medical list in that district:

The Clarke Memorial Health Centre

Dear Colleague,

I am organizing a really interesting study into the effect of the number of patients seen in surgery on the quality of the service provided. I would like to get as many GPs as possible to take part, so I hope I can count on your participation. Could you just drop me a line to let me know if you are willing.

Yours sincerely,

Two weeks later he has received two replies. One is from his partner apologizing for the fact that he is on holiday in the near future and so will not be able to take part. The other is from a 60 year-old single-handed ex-member of the GMSC who demands to know whether he is in the pay of the 'CHC or some other leftie group...'.

QUESTION 5.6

Should Dr Doolittle now:

- carry on with himself as his sample?
- decide to ask the trainers at the next trainers workshop to take part?
- approach the local GP subcommittee or LMC for their support?

The second option is a commonly practised ploy, used in the hope of attracting GPs who are in some way more committed, or likely to be keener in being involved in research projects. Dr Doolittle might similarly consider approaching College members or young practitioner groups. The two main problems are:

• There is no guarantee that these groups will be any more amenable to persuasion than the larger group, especially if the method of persuasion is as impersonal as before.
• The more highly selected the sub-group the less he would be able to generalize from his findings to the larger group. His population becomes 'GPs who are trainers in Fundless' and not 'all GPs in Fundless'.

The third option is probably the best. However, Dr Doolittle might have to rethink his approach. Rather than sending an impersonal letter it may be wiser to go and see the clerk of the LMC, or the chairman of the GP sub-committee, and suggest that the project may help to show indirectly that if list sizes were reduced so as to make surgeries smaller then services to patients might be improved, and so on.

QUESTION 5.7

Which of the following bodies might it be appropriate to approach for their views and cooperation?

- Family Health Services Authority
- District Health Authority
- District Ethical Committee

- Local Medical Committee
- Consultant Advisory Committee
- Community Health Council
- Medical Defence Union.

Dr Doolittle wants to gain the confidence and cooperation of parties representing those likely to be affected by the project in order to increase the response rate, yet he does not want this stage of the planning to drag on interminably whilst the views of committee after committee are sought.

If Dr Doolittle was surveying a large group of GPs in a district it would make sense to take his plans to any representative body that may exist such as an LMC or GP sub-committee. Similarly with the consultants. If the number to be solicited is small, then personal discussion is the best method of achieving cooperation. If the number is larger he should seek out a representative body for their views, such as the relevant Medical Advisory Committee. The Community Health Council might be thought to be at least one body which represents patients as a group. It is doubtful whether any project needs to be referred to bodies such as Health Authorities, FHSAs, or defence unions. (Though he might want the advice or cooperation of individuals, such as the Director of Public Health or FHSA managers, within such organizations.)

It is also important to spend time and effort getting people's co-operation within the practice. If there is a Patient Participation Group in the practice, perhaps they could be used as a source of opinion about the methodology chosen. Time spent in ensuring the co-operation of those helping with the data collection, both collectors and respondents, will be amply rewarded in increasing the response rate from the project and so helping to ensure the adequacy of the sample taken.

Dr Doolittle makes an appointment to see the chairman of the local LMC to elicit his support. Dr Doolittle explains to him that he would like to choose 20 GPs from Fundless Health District randomly, contact them, and persuade them to take part in his study. He points out the earlier published work suggesting that spending longer with a patient improves patient care, and suggests that if he could show that reducing the number of patients seen per surgery session, irrespective of the time spent with each patient, would improve the service provided, then that would be a strong argument for a reduction in individual list size. The chairman seems very interested but before agreeing to take the matter further asks whether Dr Doolittle has been through the ethical committee.

QUESTION 5.8

Should Dr Doolittle:

- disagree that it needs to be referred to them?
- agree to refer the project to his local ethical committee immediately?

The first option is not likely to please the chairman, and therefore Dr Doolittle might put his co-operation at risk. The second option is the proper course, but could be very time consuming. And as the research design does not directly affect patient care, it may be sufficient to discuss the project with the chairman of the local ethical committee.

The chairman of the ethical committee agrees that there are no serious ethical considerations, and that Dr Doolittle can proceed, but he requests a protocol that can be put before the committee when it next meets. (And since you are obviously so keen on research and as there is a vacancy on the ethical committee for a token GP, he invites you to be a member of that committee....)

ETHICAL CONSIDERATIONS

On the basis that any interaction with patients has the potential for harm, probably all projects involving patient opinions or details should be referred automatically to the local ethical committee. However, it is a matter for judgement, and in the not too distant past (and possibly the present in some areas) the makeup of these committees had little to do with the type of research commonly carried out in general practice. The 'District Ethical Committee' was often a sub-committee of the hospital consultants' committee structure, and almost entirely composed of this species of animal, who if certain stories are to be believed, seemed more content to allow a double-blind trial than a question to patients about what their doctors had told them. However, times are changing, and these committees are becoming far more broadly based in their composition with representation from many groups including GPs and lay members. Ethical committee approval is important to ensure that patients' interests are protected, and the committee may draw attention to problems that may have slipped unnoticed into the design of the project. It is also usually necessary to obtain such approval in any projects for which outside funding is being sought.

It should be possible to trace the whereabouts of your local ethical committee either through your postgraduate centre or library, or through the District Health Authority.

QUESTION 5.9

As a member of the local medical ethical committee Dr Doolittle has received the following protocol for a research project. What comments should he make on it, and how might it be changed to improve its chances of ethical committee approval?

Research Protocol
Title: Assessing the effect of vitamin B on the hypersensitivity of bronchial smooth muscle in primates.

It is hypothesized that hypovitaminosis may lead to a potentiation of the bronchial smooth muscles, and that eliminating such deficiencies will lessen the sensitivity of the musculature to external stimuli.

Aim: It is the aim of the project to assess the effect of regular vitamin B supplements on the peak flow readings of people known to have bronchial hypersensitivity.

Problem: The null hypothesis can be stated as: Daily supplements of vitamin B will not cause a significant increase in the early morning peak flow readings.

Details of method: Since asthma is common in young people it is proposed to look at the people in the 1–10 age group, known to have bronchial hypersensitivity. A sample of these patients will be identified from the discharge summaries of a district general hospital. No further prescriptions for anti-asthmatic treatment will be issued for a period of two weeks leading to the start of the trial to allow base-line values of peak flow to be established. Families and GPs of the patients will be sent an explanatory letter.

The sample will be divided into an intervention and a control group, matched for age and sex. The intervention group will be given vitamin B tablets, two daily, for two weeks, and the control group a placebo. Early morning peak flows will be measured in both groups. Withdrawal from the trial will be solely at the discretion of the project director, to whom application should be made.

Application: It is expected that the results will provide interesting and valuable information on the role of vitamin B on the Zartolf–Baronsky receptors in the bronchial musculature of primates.

When choosing groups to study, special care should be taken with:

- children
- unemployed
- prisoners
- pregnant women
- (• solicitors).

Some groups are easier to identify (pregnant women), or to study (prisoners). However, it is important that the vulnerability of the group be considered. Most patients trust their doctors, and may well consent to almost any proposal. It goes without saying that the doctor carries a moral responsibility for actions that are, or are not, proposed. This is more obvious in a clinical trial type of project, but may be equally important in attitudinal surveys. For pregnant women, infants, and children under 10, the requirements for informed consent are particularly stringent, and the method to be used for obtaining consent should be clearly indicated.

Similarly, the benefits that are likely to accrue from their involvement in research projects should be made clear to groups such as prisoners and their informed consent obtained. In the protocol above, one needs to ask 'Why children?' In any research using children as the study population, one should ask—can this study only be carried out on children?

QUESTION 5.10

Patients' involvement in a research project should, where possible, be preceded by:

- nothing
- verbal explanation
- written explanation
- verbal consent
- written consent.

As pointed out above, patients, for some reason, tend to trust their doctor. This means that the doctor should do everything to ensure that this trust is neither damaged nor misplaced. The words 'informed consent' imply a range of meaning, and probably hide a multitude of sins. The method of informing the patient about the project, and their involvement in it, and then the task of seeking their consent will obviously vary with the type, complexity, and implied risk of the project. The important point is that the problem must be considered properly and carefully, and an ethical committee will be looking very carefully at this part of a protocol. In the example above, there was no attempt to seek consent at any level from the parents. 'A letter of explanation' was to be sent. Yet the design of the trial was such as to put a vulnerable group, children and especially asthmatic children, at considerable risk.

QUESTION 5.11

Withdrawal from a project should be at the discretion of:

- the patient
- the project director
- the patient's doctor
- the ethical committee.

Withdrawal from a project of any type, at any stage, must remain the right of the patient. Similarly any doctor must remain free to remove a patient under his or her care from a project, especially a trial, or to give additional treatment at any time, if it seems to be in the patient's best interests. In the example, withdrawal from a dangerous trial was to be at the discretion of the project director—an obviously unrealistic and unethical approach.

In summary, it is important to consider the ethical issues implicit in the design of any project.

One needs to ask:

- Is the research necessary? Will it have positive applications for future health care?

• Will the research project be well planned and executed? It is unethical to carry out any project that is not.
• If the trial or project involves children, is it of such a nature that it can only be carried out on children?
• Has the informed consent of the patient, or the parent, been obtained, before their participation and before randomization?
• Is it clear that patients are free to withdraw from the trial at any time if they so wish?
• Is it clear that any doctor responsible for the care of the patient is free to remove that patient from the trial, or to give additional treatment at any time, if he or she feels it to be in the patient's best interests?
• Is the project to be controlled and supervised by a properly constituted ethical committee?

Hopefully, this has given you some idea of the areas covered by ethical considerations of projects and trials. The WHO has produced the Helsinki Declaration on the subject, the main points of which can be found in a medical library.

Dr Doolittle returns to the problem of finding 20 doctors to take part in his plan. The chairman of the LMC is also now satisfied and so he selects a random sample of twenty GPs from the medical list for Fundless.

QUESTION 5.12

The chairman of the LMC suggests to Dr Doolittle that they send a joint letter to these doctors asking them to participate.
Should Dr Doolittle agree?

Yes? Despite the extra weight of the LMC sanction, a written request may only produce a small increase on the initial letter.

No? Dr Doolittle tactfully suggests that the LMC chairman writes a letter that he can then show the GPs when he goes and visits them to explain the project, and to try and persuade them to participate.

Using a table of random numbers and the local medical list, he identifies his sample of twenty doctors. He makes appointments to see them all, and explain the outline of the project, why they have been chosen, the backing of the local LMC, and the likely consequences from the results.

QUESTION 5.13

Despite this, eight of the twenty decide not to take part. Should Dr Doolittle:
• accuse them of anti-social behaviour and report them to the GMC?
• make up the number from among his own partners, trainees, and colleagues?

- take another eight names from the list using the list of random numbers, and contact these as before?

The first option has its appeal, but sticking pins into effigies is probably just as effective.

The second option would mean that the sample was no longer random. However, with eight out of twenty refusing to take part for whatever reason there are going to be doubts about the randomness of the sample whichever method is chosen. This is probably not the best alternative, though it may be the most practical.

The third option is probably the most correct thing to do. However, based on the previous drop-out rate, only four of these may be willing to take part, and it may be that by the time twenty places have been filled Dr Doolittle will have approached almost half his possible population (with all the work this will entail).

QUESTION 5.14

What should Dr Doolittle do about the drop-outs?

- ignore them as unscientific doctors
- record information about them for future use!

Much as Dr Doolittle would like to, he cannot ignore them as there may be something different about this sizeable sub-group—quite separate from their non-compliance with research invitations.

The second option may appear to contain a touch of 'big brother', but in fact he will need to know whether this group of non-responders differs in any way from his responding GPs. That is, is there anything different about them such that findings from the responding GPs would not apply equally to these non-responders? To that end he will need to record the characteristics of his non-responders to compare them with his responders in the analysis.

INTERVIEWING

Dr Sophie Middleyear decides to look at the connection between symptoms associated with the so-called 'male menopause' as well as female menopause, and life events. She designs a questionnaire to be put to a sample of her patients aged between 40 and 55. She feels that an interview will be a more effective way of eliciting information than a postal questionnaire, but because of resource limitations she has to carry out some of the interviewing herself. Although she has never done any interviewing before she does not envisage any problems. After all, she spends most of her day talking to patients, and interviewing is only a matter of establishing and recording the information she needs. So off she goes to find some patients with a bunch of questionnaires in her hand, and a pencil behind her ear.

But hold on. How does she find a sample of respondents? Chapter 2 described how random sampling would enable her to limit the size of her project without necessarily affecting the meaningfulness of the results. Therefore she identifies the 50 names and addresses of a sample of 40–55-year-old patients from the practice age–sex register. She has a young trainee who is keen to help her (and perhaps even keener to get a good reference!). How does she select the ones that she will approach, and those the other interviewer will attempt to contact?

QUESTION 5.15

Should Dr Middleyear pick out:

- patients whom she knows will be friendly?
- patients who live in certain affluent areas because she finds poorer people a bit stroppy?
- male patients as she finds female patients a bit difficult?
- all patients in a certain area?

All interviewers should try and interview a cross section of the sample, so the first two options should not be used. However, there are limitations to time and resources, and it would seem wise to allocate addresses in the same locality to each interviewer.

The first name on Dr Middleyear's list is:

Mrs Olive Wintergreen
83 The Walk
Little Puddle-on-Sea

Her knock is answered by a Mr Biggs who tells her that Mrs Wintergreen no longer lives there.

QUESTION 5.16

Should Dr Middleyear:

- finish the interview there and then?
- interview Mr Biggs?
- ask for Mrs Wintergreen's new address?

The third option is the most rigorous course of action, but a decision has to be made about how far movers should be followed up. More expediently, some studies use a procedure where a substitute is picked. This is acceptable so long as the randomness of the sample is not compromised.

The next name and address on her list is:

Mr A. Daly
Warrick Mansion
The Hill
Little Puddle-on-Sea

When Dr Middleyear gets there she gets no reply and the house looks suspiciously vacant and derelict.

QUESTION 5.17

Apart from rushing to see her bank manager to buy it and turn it into an old people's home, should she:

- ask the neighbours where Mr Daly has moved to?
- call back later, just in case he is out?
- give up and send a postal questionnaire?

Occasionally the house really will be derelict or vacant. Interviewers can then ask neighbours to see where the occupants have moved to. On other occasions the respondents will just be out at the time the interviewer calls. In such cases the interviewer will usually make up to three visits before a decision is made to give up the attempt at gaining an interview.

Obtaining an interview

Disheartened, Dr Middleyear wonders if she should have done a project on housing. Where is everyone this warm summer day?
    She moves on to the third name and address on her list hoping for more luck.

Mrs Pamela Croucher
2, Battle Drive
Greater Puddle-on-Sea

Eureka! The lady in question is at home. So Dr Middleyear gives her the basic information about the survey, its relevance, and why she has been selected. Despite this she seems very reluctant to take part.

QUESTION 5.18

Should Dr Middleyear:

- give up and accept the refusal?
- tell her that she is being unco-operative and threaten to strike her off her list?
- gently persuade her to take part?

One of the most difficult but crucial steps is to get the respondent to agree to be interviewed. Increasingly, people are wary of strangers appearing on door-steps asking them to divulge information about their private lives. Obviously the second option would never be used because every respondent has the right to refuse and it is up to the interviewer to put a reasonable case rather than tell the respondent he or she is in some way morally wrong not to take part in the vitally important research. Much will depend on the strength of a respondent's feelings about being interviewed. Perhaps giving up and accepting the refusal is the right course; however, in some cases gentle persuasion is possible.

QUESTION 5.19

Spend a few minutes thinking of the points that could be made in an attempt to gently persuade Mrs Croucher to take part.

It may purely be a question of convenience—offering to return at a more convenient time may be all that is needed. It could be that she does not fully understand why she has been picked out (is there something wrong with her?), and so by emphasizing the random structure of the sampling and her selection, and by fully and clearly explaining the importance of gaining an interview with her, she may change her mind. It is possible that she does not know who the interviewer is, and this may especially be the case if other helpers are used— some form of identification might help. Some of this uncertainty can be overcome by sending a letter to the sample before beginning the study, telling them about it and asking for their co-operation. The respondent then has the option of contacting the researcher directly to find out more about the study or to refuse to take part, thereby not wasting travelling time. However, sending a letter has the danger of encouraging refusals and in general face-to-face contact between interviewer and respondent is a better way of gaining co-operation than more formal means such as a letter.

Asking the questions

Pamela eventually lets Dr Middleyear in and gives her a cup of tea. She settles down to ask the questions.

After the first few questions it becomes clear that Mrs Croucher's responses, particularly with the open-ended questions, are unclear, incomplete, and irrelevant.

QUESTION 5.20

Should Dr Middleyear:

* accept what is said and write it down verbatim?
* ignore the unclear replies and move on to the next question?

- avoid and omit open-ended questions?
- clarify the answer for the respondent?
- allow for an expectant pause?
- encourage a response, e.g. 'that's interesting'?
- repeat the question?
- use a supplementary question or probe for clarification: 'I'm not quite sure what you mean'?
- add neutral comments such as 'anything else?'?

The last six options are accepted procedures used by trained interviewers to elicit full responses to questions. Thus, it may be helpful to sit down with the trainee, or other helpers, before starting, to go over the questions and their meanings. This may also be the time to point out that the success from such interviews can also depend on the tone of voice, manner, gesture, and personal characteristics of the interviewer, as well as the circumstances under which the interview is carried out. Depending on the type and subject matter of the questions, it might be possible to maximize the success of the survey by recruiting helpers to interview according to age, social class, gender, and so on.

After three hours with Mrs Croucher and with only three of the 46 questions answered—and for two of those the still confused replies were only extracted after the shedding of much blood, sweat, and tears—Dr Middleyear decides to pass over this part of the project totally to her trainee.

CONFIDENTIALITY AND DATA PROTECTION

Research projects involve the collection and analysis of some form of data. The study of health care usually involves information about individuals, whether they be patients, doctors, or other health care workers. This information may be about the individuals or may consist of their opinions about various issues. Much of it will only be given freely by that individual if they are convinced about the confidentiality of their contributions. Confidentiality can be threatened both in the collection and in the analysis of the research data. Often confidentiality can be put at risk, unbeknown to the patients concerned, through the research method chosen.

Dr John Batter has decided to analyse the effect of intervention by the health visitor in families in which it is suspected a non-accidental injury has occurred to a child. A review of the families' medical records is undertaken to assess subsequent health problems in members of these families.

QUESTION 5.21

Who should Dr Batter ask to search the records to record the information:

- the practice secretary
- the temporarily attached research worker

- the practice attached health visitor
- the GP.

It is common knowledge, and indeed common practice in these days of primary health care teams, that access to patient records is not totally and absolutely restricted to the patient's doctor. In the daily running of a practice the notes are handled by an assortment of clerks, receptionists, secretaries, nurses, health visitors, and so on. Running a research project that involves the perusal of patient records lays open these records to more people, with resultant loss of confidentiality. Even if the subject matter is not as sensitive as in the example here, a search through records may inadvertently reveal information that was only given initially on the assumption that doctor–patient confidentiality was assured. Such searches should, in an ideal world, only be undertaken by the doctor. However, once again, economy of time and effort may demand less than the ideal, and any resulting compromise should be arrived at only after the most careful consideration of aspects of confidentiality.

Having collected the data there are still problems of confidentiality in the method chosen to store the data. A great pile of scraps of paper will obviously not be easy to analyse, and the degree of confidentiality it affords will be dependent on the researcher's ability to keep the scraps together, and to prevent unauthorized access to them.

Computerized databases are extremely common nowadays. They are relatively easy to use, both to store the data in whatever way is required, and to allow it to be presented in a form suitable for analysis. They are also perceived by both public and government as being considerably less than perfect in protecting the confidentiality of data about individuals. It is all too easy to ask a computer, assuming it stores such details, to produce a list of one-legged homosexuals working as security officers in the north-west of Scotland. Newspaper stories of computer enthusiasts 'hacking' their way into private computer mailboxes, or into the Pentagon's main computer, have somewhat dented the faith in the various 'password' methods that are meant to protect computer-held information from unauthorized prying eyes.

The Data Protection Act requires anyone who is storing patient details electronically to register their use of a computer for this purpose. Universities and research institutes will be able to advise you on this, but as they will probably already have a 'blanket' registration under the Act you may be able to carry out your research under the aegis of such arrangements.

Probably the practical compromise most commonly used in data storage is to store data with a code number as a patient identifier. The key that links code number to patient name can be kept separately. Indeed, in cases in which respondent anonymity (as well as confidentiality) is important, the key can be kept by a third party. Questionnaires are given a code number and sent out by the third party to all the people on the list, but they are returned to the researcher. It is then a simple task to ask the key holder to send out second questionnaires to the code numbers of those who failed to return the first. With this method, one person knows respondents' identities and another their actual responses, but neither can link both pieces of information.

SUMMARY

This chapter has attempted to look at various practical considerations in the carrying out of any project. Although doing research, of whatever complexity, can be extremely rewarding and enjoyable, it does require the use of resources. It is therefore extremely important that these resources are used efficiently and effect-ively. The major resource will be your energy. Be reassured that almost all researchers at some point in almost all research studies wonder why they started this particular project; but the feeling does pass! By careful planning in the form of a clearly presented research design and a rigorous pilot study you should help minimize these crises of confidence.

Also remember that probably the most precious resource that needs to be nurtured and treated with great consideration are the patients, colleagues, partners, and staff whose co-operation you will be seeking not just for the present project, but possibly again in the not too distant future.

SUGGESTED TASK

Find out the composition and procedures of your local ethical committee. How often does it meet? What percentage of applications are turned down, or are requested to be changed?

6 Data into numbers

Chapter 4 described how data could be collected and Chapter 5 described some of the practical difficulties of actually doing that collecting. It is now time to retire to your inner sanctum excitedly clutching your data. Analysis! Results! Publications! An OBE?

But look at your data: a pile of questionnaires? A collection of tape cassettes? A jumble of field notes? How are these to be analysed to produce those heady 'results'? This chapter examines the first stage in that process (mainly in so far as it relates to quantitative studies), namely the procedures by which newly collected data are transformed into numbers.

A NOTE ON QUALITATIVE METHODS

Chapter 4 outlined the overall process of collecting specific data from the mass of data 'out there'. These data could be collected by unstructured, semi-structured, and structured means and each of these forms of data require different treatments to enable analysable results to emerge.

Some unstructured data can be analysed without recourse to numbers. Inteviews with patients on the meanings they ascribe to their illnesses, for example, might be analysed in terms of the variety and types of interpretation used. Certainly this form of data could be converted into numbers—as will be shown—but almost inevitably with some loss of quality. Although analysing numbers is the traditional way of doing research, it is increasingly recognized that qualitative studies have an important role to play in reaching a deeper under-standing of phenomena. A structured questionnaire given to receptionists to ascertain their views of patients might give some numbers to play with, but a few in-depth interviews may reveal far more of interest than would a thousand fixed format questionnaires.

This chapter concentrates on quantitative research to the extent that the end-product is numbers, but this is not to imply that it is necessarily superior. It all depends on what you are trying to do. If the research question is about whether winter-born children are more likely to develop URTIs during the rest of their childhoods then this must be a quantitative study. But if you want to know how the child's parents cope with these infections you might find a qualitative study of greater value. General practice remains a little-researched and in many ways little-understood area, and different approaches all have an important part to play in its exploration. A summary of how data can be analysed without recourse to numbers is given in the final section of the chapter.

QUANTITATIVE STUDIES

Let us first take an overview of the rest of the research process after data collection.

1. Data are converted into numbers.
2. Numbers will need to be analysed by manipulation (Chapter 7) and usually with some form of statistical summary (Chapter 9).
3. Results will be written up (Chapter 10).

The analysis will probably be carried out using a computer, either a large computer or powerful network as is found in universities—gaining access by a 'terminal'—or by a stand-alone personal computer (as might be found in a general practice). Increasingly the power of personal computers is such that they can tackle most analyses, even sophisticated statistical manipulations of data, that might be needed on general practice data. There are a number of commercial software packages available to carry out these analyses, but a good alternative—and free, because it is in the public domain—is Epi Info. Details of using this package come later in Chapter 8. In the meantime any data will need organizing into a form that makes them easy to analyse.

THE DATA FILE

Computers need to 'read' numbers in an assimilable form: this is the 'data file' (a file being a discrete collection of information stored in a computer, analogous to a file in a filing cabinet).

Dr Verity Tally is interested in exploring the patterns of work in her consultations. She collects data on all the patients she sees during a week, together with information on whether she wrote a prescription or referred for investigation or an outpatient appointment. She sees 130 patients in the week and collects the relevant data on a schedule, in the form of an audit sheet, which she designed specially for the purpose. She then processes her data into a data file, the first five lines of which look like this:

$$0016922111$$
$$0025411112$$
$$0034322111$$
$$0042321111$$
$$0053212211$$

What does it all mean? Fortunately Dr Tally knows, and she will let the computer into the secret so that it too can 'read' the data file.

The data file is a series of columns running downwards and rows running across. Looking down the left-hand three columns, you should be able to see a pattern. Each set of three digits is a number, ascending from one line to the next. This is because each line or row represents one 'case'—one patient who was seen by Dr Tally in her survey week. In this example each case is ten digits long, but in other studies it might be longer or shorter depending on how much data on each have been collected. (Sometimes computers can only cope with a maximum line length of 80 digits, but each case can, if needed, take up several lines.)

Let us explore what each line means. Take the first one:

0016922111

Although it might look like either ten separate numbers or one large one, it is in fact several groups of numbers. In this example Dr Tally knows that the digits break up into the following groups:

001 69 2 2 1 1 1

The first three columns contain the case number. In this instance it is 001. The case number requires three digits because, as you will recall, Dr Tally collected 130 patients in her audit. Had she collected a sample of 9 or fewer, then one column would have sufficed; on the other hand if her sample had been over 999 then she would have required four columns/digits, the first case becoming 0001.

The next two columns contain the patient's age. This is very straightforward. It is clear that the first patient was 69; equally going back to the data file it can be seen that the second was 54, and so on.

Dr Tally reserved the sixth column for the patient's sex. Dr Tally started off with two possibilities, male or female. But the computer does not read words as part of the English language so Dr Tally has to devise a *code* to represent the two sexes to the computer. The code could be groups of letters such as MALE or FEMALE but this is rather cumbersome as well as wasteful. The more usual way of coding is to assign one number or letter to each category. This could have been:

male   = M
female = F.

The letters have the advantage of being fairly easily recognizable, but also the slight disadvantage that computers often find numbers less cumbersome and easier to manipulate. Thus, in this case Dr Tally chose:

male   = 1
female = 2.

Thus knowing the code, it can be seen that the first patient she recorded was a 69-year-old female.

In similar fashion the next four columns are reserved for codes of practice activity. The coding system that Dr Tally chose was:

Column 7   Prescription?   no = 1
                                  yes = 2

Column 8	X-ray?	no = 1
		yes = 2
Column 9	Pathology	no = 1
		yes = 2
Column 10	OP referral?	no = 1
		yes = 2

Now reading along the data line it can be seen that the first patient in the audit was a 69-year-old woman who received a prescription but was not referred for an X-ray, for pathology investigation, or to outpatients.

It all begins to make sense. Which patient was referred to outpatients? The second, because there is a figure 2 in the tenth column. Which was the youngest patient to receive a prescription? The fifth, who was 32. (The fourth was the youngest at 23, but the figure 1 in the sixth column indicates that no prescription was issued.)

For a small number of cases (or small data set, to use the technical term) the data file can be read 'manually'. However, with the full data file of 130 cases, reading this sort of data off visually becomes a chore, even more so with hundreds of cases and perhaps 80 columns of data for each. But this sort of task is precisely what computers are good at. So long as the computer knows the code, it can read off whatever information is required. Moreover, the computer can manipulate the data. It can be asked, for example, to add all the ages and divide by the number of cases to produce an average (mean) age. It can calculate the percentage of patients receiving prescriptions by adding the 2s in the seventh column and expressing the result as a percentage of all the cases. And, more interestingly, it can compare some cases with others: are women, for instance, more likely to receive prescriptions than men? (Which are the women? Read column six. Which of those received prescriptions? Read column seven. Compare this result with the figures for men. And so on.) This manipulation of numbers in the data file will be more fully explored in the next two chapters.

The first task, however, is to translate any data that has been collected into a computer-readable format, as above. How is this done? Basically, it depends on the degree to which the collected data has already been categorized. The simplest type of data to transform into a data file are structured data, while the most complicated are unstructured. (The reasons why this is so were given in Chapter 4.) Let us start with the easier task: structured data.

STRUCTURED SCHEDULES

Chapter 4 described three types of structured schedule: a clinical schedule, an extraction schedule, and a traditional questionnaire. There was a similar format in all of these:

closed question $\Rightarrow$ answer

A series of closed questions were answered by the respondent or interviewer in fixed format. The answer format is relatively fixed because the closed question ensured this was so. Thus, it can reasonably be assumed that a question about height in metres will not be answered in terms of weight, or, hopefully, in units other than metres.

The task of transforming responses into numbers is therefore a relatively straightforward one. The pile of questionnaires/schedules has to be *coded,* that is the set responses have to be transcribed into numbers and entered into a data file as described above.

Let us look at some general points about coding. The process goes like this:

responses on ⇒ numbers on ⇒ data file
schedule   data sheet   in computer

The traditional way of transforming numbers into the computer was by first 'punching' holes at appropriate places on a special data card using a special sort of typewriter. Each case had a separate card. These cards were then 'read' by a machine and the data automatically entered into the computer. With the advent of the personal computer this process has been shortened by cutting out the card stage and entering data directly into the computer using the number key pad usually found on standard keyboards. Even so, although numbers are now entered directly, the old expression of 'punching' data is still often used to describe this process.

Punching large quantities of data into a computer can be a chore and if your data are extensive you might find it worthwhile to pay to have it done by technicians who are as fast at typing numbers as secretaries are at typing letters. (Ask about this facility at your local university department of general practice.) If you do want to do it yourself, you could use a wordprocessor to type the numbers in as an unformatted document or get the program to create an ASCII file. (An ASCII file is a basic data file without the embedded formatting commands that wordprocessors usually insert). This can be read as a data file either by statistical software you might use yourself or by the software used by more complex larger computers.

Coding formats

How does Dr Tally code her audit? In part it depends on how she recorded her data. Let us look at two formats she might have used.

Number	Age	Sex	Prescription	X-ray	Path.	OP
001	69	F				
002	54	M				
003	43	F				

This first format, which records all the data on to one sheet, might need some intermediate steps before it is punched. There might be a data sheet, a separate sheet of paper on which are written the appropriate numbers based on the coding frame described earlier. The endpoint would be a handwritten data file which would then be punched onto the computer. The alternative—as the data are relatively straightforward—is to punch it in directly, doing the coding as the original data are read. Thus, Dr Tally could run her finger along one line of data, code it in her head and punch it out on the keyboard with her other hand. This technique cuts out the separate data sheet, and would therefore seem more efficient. However, it means that you are likely to have to do the punching yourself as trained punchers tend to work only from data sheets. (Quite reasonably they cannot be expected to memorize the proper codings for every piece of data set that they punch in.)

The other common format in which data are collected is to have a separate sheet for every case. In Dr Tally's project it might look like this:

Audit sheet

Number
Age
Sex (M/F)
Prescription
X-ray
Pathology
OP Referral

Here again, as with the earlier example, data can be directly punched or first transcribed on to a data sheet. There is a short-cut to the latter procedure, however, because the space on the schedule allows us to place the data sheet on the same piece of paper. Thus:

Audit sheet

| | For office |
| | use only |

Number
Age
Sex (M/F)
Prescription
X-ray
Pathology
OP Referral

A margin down the right-hand side of the paper bears a threatening heading such as 'Office use only' or 'Please do not write in this margin'. The reason for keeping it clear is to allow the actual numbers for the data file to be written in. Moreover the boxes for the data file numbers can be annotated with the numbers of the column in which the data are to be entered. (Though notice boxes/columns 1–5 do not require transcribing as the researcher or respondent enters the actual number directly onto the schedule.) Using this technique, especially when there are lots of data per case, the puncher can keep an accurate check on which column each digit goes into.

The final piece of the jigsaw is for the coder to have a coding sheet, describing the numbers which will represent whatever answers are on the sheet. In Dr Tally's project it might look something like this:

Coding sheet for audit

Columns			
1–3	Number		
4–5	Age		
6	Sex	male = 1	female = 2
7	Prescription		
8	X-ray		no = 1
9	Pathology		yes = 2
10	OP referral		

If each member of her family has a pen and a coding sheet, and is willing to help, Dr Tally would be able to pile her schedules on the kitchen table and quickly code her 130 cases.

Coding conventions

There are several conventions in coding, none of which are vital to follow, but which show good sense and order; you may like to copy them.

Make the actual number the code

In Dr Tally's coding sheet she did not give a separate code for the case number. If she had felt creative she could have multiplied the case number by three and used that number: possible but silly. Clearly the sensible thing with many numbers is to code them directly: height, weight, diastolic pressure, for example, can all be punched. without change

Categorize clumsy numbers or those in which precision is doubtful

Patient's height (metres) $\boxed{1.43521}$

Sometimes the researcher or the respondent gives too much detail. A height given to a fraction of a millimetre is not worth coding complete unless the research was particularly concerned with very fine variations in height.

The customary technique in science is to 'round up or down'. This in fact is a sort of categorization because if it is decided that height is only needed to the nearest centimetre then the coding rule is:

$$1.465–1.474 = 1.47$$
$$1.475–1.484 = 1.48$$
$$1.485–1.494 = 1.49$$

In this case, the above example would be coded as 1.48 because it falls into this category.

This principle can be extended to group any kind of data. For example, Dr Tally coded age as the actual age in years. She might however have decided that she was only interested in ten-year age bands and thus her coding rule might have looked like this:

under 20 = 1
20–29   = 2
30–39   = 3
40–49   = 4
50–59   = 5
60–69   = 6
over 69 = 7

Using this schema her first patient, the 69- year-old woman would have scored 7 for her age (and Dr Tally would have needed one less column in her data file).

Alternatively Dr Tally might only have been interested in her elderly population. She could thus have devised a dichotomous scale:

under 65   = 1
65 and over = 2

Her first patient would then have scored 2. Clearly the categories employed will depend on the precise research question, and the coding scheme for age in one study might be completely inappropriate for another. A word of caution though. Dr Tally might have started out being interested in her prescribing rate amongst her elderly patients compared with her younger patients and therefore coded either 1 or 2 for age. However, if she finds higher prescribing amongst her elderly and wonders whether perhaps there is a linear relationship between age and prescribing such that the older you are the more prescriptions you get, she cannot test this on her data: remember, she 'lost' her precise age data by only coding it 1 or 2. A wiser course of action—if resources and space permits—is to code numbers as completely as possible. Dr Tally could then ask the computer to split her sample into 'young' and 'elderly' for her research question and, if she wants to go back to the original ages, she can ask the computer to split them again into their original ages as given in the data file.

Coding non-integer data

Frequently, collected data are on a dichotomous scale, e.g. drug/not drug, consulted/not consulted, and here a simple 1/2 will suffice as the code. Other data will be in the form of a number that can be transcribed as outlined above. Yet other data will have no clear mathematical transformation and in these cases codes can be assigned arbitrarily. For example:

$$
\begin{array}{ll}
\text{Protestant} & = 1 \\
\text{Catholic} & = 2 \\
\text{Jew} & = 3 \\
\text{Other} & = 4
\end{array}
$$

Religious affiliation might be coded as above; or it might be coded 4, 3, 2, 1 or 3, 1, 2, 4. It really doesn't matter. So long as particular religious groups are coded consistently with the same code number and the computer is told what that code is, then it can all be sorted out later.

Missing answers, don't knows, spoiled replies

Not infrequently, especially in self-administered questionnaires, data are incomplete. Respondents might simply omit to answer a question; or they might answer it inappropriately. Sometimes whole questionnaires have to be rejected because of this and the respondent placed in the non-response category as if they had declined to take part in the study. Often, however, some questions are answered appropriately but others need a little thought before coding

QUESTION 6.1

How would you code the following responses?

1. Are you male or female?   male ☐ *cheeky!*
      (please tick)   female ☐
2. Are you male or female?   male ☐
      (please tick)   female ☐
3. Are you male or female?   male ☐
      (please tick)   female ☐ *woman*
4. Are you male or female?   male ☒
      (please tick)   female ☐

1. Not the most helpful of respondents. In a survey of transsexuals this response might be taken seriously and be given its own code, say 3, but in this instance it would count as a spoiled answer and, following a common convention which reserves 9 for missing answers, can be coded 9.

2. The question was simply not answered. It cannot therefore be coded either 1 or 2. It must therefore be scored as missing with a 9.

3. Not answered precisely as was requested but it would seem reasonable to code this respondent as female, 2.

4. A tick was requested in the appropriate box but here 'male' was marked with a cross. Was the cross a substitute for a tick? Or does it signify 'not' male? There is no absolute way of telling, but a look at other responses in the questionnaire

might suggest whether this respondent was consistently using a cross instead of a tick.

UNSTRUCTURED AND SEMI-STRUCTURED SCHEDULES

The process described above involved devising a 'coding rule' which enabled responses to be transformed into standardized numbers. Thus the response 'male/female' was transformed into 1/2 by the coding rule male = 1, female = 2. Coding an unstructured or semi-structured schedule follows exactly the same logical process, but because of the variability in the format of the response the coding rules must be that much more complex.

Let us look at a relatively straightforward example from a semi-structured schedule and then a more complicated one from an unstructured schedule.

Semi-structured schedules

Dr John Pole has been conducting a survey of patient satisfaction with his services. He has persuaded his local Community Health Council to interview a random sample of his patients. One of the questions is an open-ended one:

How satisfied are you with Dr Pole as your GP?

The interviewers from the CHC wrote down verbatim the patient's replies. Here are a some of them:

A. He's an excellent doctor.

B. He can be a bit rude at times but he was spot on with George's arthritis.

C. I've never met him.

D. I always use the other partners.

E. He always comes when I call him out.

F. He's a terrible doctor ... I always avoid him.

G. My diabetes has been a real worry ... then there was Mary's cough ... drove me round the bend ... the medicine didn't work though it's not his fault.

H. I get on with him though I know people who don't.

If Dr Pole had asked a closed question it might have been of this form

Are you satisfied with your GP?	yes ❑
(Please tick)	no ❑
	indifferent ❑

This could have been easily coded 1, 2, or 3. This same logic can be applied to the open-ended question to score a similar 1, 2, or 3. The coding rule might be something like this:

Does the patient make positive comments?	then = 1
Does the patient make negative comments?	then = 2
Is it unclear whether comments are on balance positive or negative then = 3	

Using this schema respondents A and E only have good things to say and would be scored 1. Respondent F is clearly negative and would score 2. Respondent B does make a passing negative comment but strongly qualifies it with a positive one. It would seem reasonable to score it 1. Respondent C has never met him so must be a 3. Respondent D's comment could be a negative one—perhaps he uses the other partners to avoid our doctor—but it is not clear. A middle of the road 3 would probably be appropriate here. Respondent G is loquacious but while skirting close to criticizing the doctor ('the medicine didn't work') denies the opportunity of making a critical remark. Certainly not a 2. Possibly that can be seen as a 'reluctantly' positive response and score a 1, or, being very cautious, a 3. Likewise respondent H gives two different opinions; but as the assessment is of the respondent's own view it would seem right to score 1.

In this way the same sort of result as would be obtained from a closed question might result. Why not therefore use a closed question—it would certainly be easier? Mainly because it is believed that the *quality* of the responses is better. Respondent B might have simply thought of the doctor's occasional rudeness and ticked the 'not satisfied' box, whereas it seems that the actual view is more easily balanced if not on the positive side. And so on. Taking this argument further means that if more 'talk' is elicited from respondents then the better the quality of the final scores.

In the example above, data were lost by classifying responses into three boxes: the ambivalence of B was lost, as was the diabetes and cough in G's account. In short, coding involves 'data reduction' and of necessity misses the subtleties of the different ways patients arrived at an assessment of their doctor. Of course, in collapsing all those words into numbers there were bound to be lost data, although the loss might not be as great if the coding system had been more sophisticated. For example, in the coding there could have been separate scores for patient satisfaction with the GP's personal manner and with his clinical competence (to be entered in two separate columns in the data file). Thus, respondent B would score a 2 on the interpersonal satisfaction scale yet a 1 on the clinical satisfaction scale; respondent H would score a 1 on the interpersonal and a 3 (for don't know/indifferent) on the clinical.

An alternative strategy for squeezing more and better quality scores from the data would be to extend the satisfaction scales. Respondent A would seem to be far more glowing about the GP than H and yet with a dichotomous scale both would score a 1 for being satisfied. The following coding frame might encompass this:

Strongly positive comments = 1
Positive comments   = 2
Neither positive nor negative = 3
Negative comments   = 4
Strongly negative comments = 5

In this schema, A would be a 1 and H a 2 while F would be a 5 and so on. If the data warranted it the scale could be widened even further and/or other sub-scales created for different dimensions of satisfaction. Inevitably, this process is limited by the quantity and quality of the 'talk data' collected. In this case only one comment was recorded for each respondent, but knowing what the coding scheme is, it would have been possible to guide the interviews to cover precisely these areas. Otherwise, if the coding system is too elaborate and the data are flimsy, most respondents will end up in the 'unknown' category. Nevertheless, the general principle is an important one and had the respondents been encouraged to talk more of their GP then more sophisticated coding frames would have been possible.

Remember that whereas coding frames for structured schedules can be devised *before* data are collected (because the limits of the answers are known), in the case of more open-ended questions the data must be seen before appropriate frames can be devised. One way round this problem is to create the frame on data collected in a pilot survey so that everything is prepared when data from the main study come rolling in.

Unstructured schedules

The general principle of using some 'rules' to convert qualitative data into quantitative can be seen further in the analysis of 'talk data' such as a tape-recorded interview using an unstructured or semi-structured questionnaire. Here it is possible to look for much more subtle things than would be possible using structured techniques.

Dr Enid Hart believes that the worst cases of rheumatoid arthritis are found in women with poor self-esteem. (Wisely, she declines to put a causal inference on the observation as it could be in either direction: RA might cause loss of self-esteem just as low self-esteem might cause RA.) She decides to use the quantity of analgesics consumed as an indicator of the severity of the RA for the patient. For self-esteem she interviews the women and tapes the conversation: she asks each about their lives and feelings of self-worth; the tapes last up to an hour. Back in her study the pile of cassettes grows. The time has come to analyse them before other members of the family sabotage the research by replacing her data with Barry Manilow. Trapped amongst all the words recorded on the tapes is the respondents' self-esteem. How can it be extracted?

Rating scales

First Dr Hart must decide precisely what she is looking for. What is self-esteem exactly? If she doesn't know what it is she is hardly likely to find it. Thus the first task is both to define self-esteem and from the definition construct a *rating scale* that will act as a sort of template for scoring her patients. (In effect she is taking a 'concept' and operationalizing it; see Chapter 3.)

After much discussion with friends, and reading and thinking, Dr Hart decides that there are probably three components to self-esteem, namely:

- feelings of value about one's body
- feelings of worth about one's mind/personality
- perceived quality of relationship with others

Each of these components will need teasing out; furthermore, each component will need scoring on a scale. The length of this scale will depend on both the richness of the concept, in other words Dr Hart's ability to distinguish different degrees of self-worth, and the richness of the data on cassette tape; will they be subtle enough to enable assignment to one of the points on the scale, or indeed to the scale itself.

Dr Hart discusses 'feelings of value about one's own body' with her colleagues. They agree that there must be a point at either end of the scale to represent either extreme pride and contentment in physical appearance or the absolute opposite. In between is more difficult. One of her colleagues points out that his feelings of worth vary—if he is well dressed he feels good; another colleague says he feels awful after getting up and is glad there is no one there to see him. Dr Hart is beginning to get some points for her rating scale:

Always feeling one's body looks good	= 1
Some ambivalence about features of one's body but a feeling that these can be overcome with cosmetics, clothes, a good tan, etc.	= 2
Constant concern about some aspects of body, though relatively minor	= 3
More serious concern about body, of sufficient severity to affect interaction	= 4
Periodic bouts of feeling one's body is ugly	= 5
Always feel one is unattractive	= 6

It is important that Dr Hart's colleagues have helped devise this 'rating scale' because she will need them to help her by being 'raters'. It is obvious that raters must be very familiar with the scale they are using if they are all to use it consistently. Had Dr Hart devised the scale entirely on her own she would have had to 'teach' it to her colleagues and then ensure that they all had the same ideas by testing it on some pilot data.

QUESTION 6.2

Having devised the above rating scale on body perception, Dr Hart wants to try it out. As one of her raters, how would you score the following transcripts taken from interviews recorded on tape. (Ideally you would listen to the tape itself in case tone of voice, pauses, and so on, helped you in your ratings.)

W: Since I was a little girl I have known I had a weight problem ... it's just that nothing seems to fit ... it's probably because I like my food so much ... I find it so difficult to cut down ... the children don't help, they're constantly wanting cakes and things ... mind you I'm getting to the point when it's hardly worth bothering with ... at my age, you know ... the only thing I worry about is diabetes ... my mother had it and they say it was her weight that did it ... she was a big woman ...

X: you wouldn't believe it now but I won a beauty contest when I was seventeen ... and in those days it was all natural, not paint and dyed hair like the young people today ... my husband said that my hair was my best feature ... it used to be very long, but its just inconvenient to have it like that now, always getting in the way ... my daughter's got long hair but she is young ... it's really lovely on her ...

Y: I've been told that I've got a lop-sided face (laughs) ... but I can't be perfect all over ... size of nose indicates character I say ... besides its never done me any harm ... I've got a wonderful family and job so I leave the looks to those who are not so fortunate ... anyway a smile gets you through any day.

Z: I never let my husband see me without make-up on ... I look dreadful ... first thing in the morning it's a real struggle ... its difficult to hide puffy eyes and wrinkles but by mid-morning I start to come alive ... some people are best in the morning, some in the evening I always say and I am an evening person ... I suppose that if I went to bed early enough I wouldn't be so bad in the morning but then I'd miss the time I like the best.

These brief excerpts from the interviews have already been scored by three raters:

	W	X	Y	Z
Rater 1	4	2	2	4
Rater 2	3	1	2	3
Rater 3	3	2	2	4
Rater 4				

Add your scores to the table as rater 4. You will note that all the scores are not exactly the same for each respondent, but they are all similar, so it suggests that something consistent is being picked out from the interviews.

Because the raters have each been 'trained' to apply the same rating scale, it can be assumed that the same measure is being applied every time a score is decided. Referring back to Chapter 3 on measuring things you will recall that the consistency of scores is a measure of the reliability of the test, in this case the application of a rating scale. In fact this characteristic of the rating scale has a special name, *inter-rater reliability*, and a special statistic associated with it (kappa) which gives a figure of 0 to 1: the closer the figure is to 1 then the more reliable our application of the rating scale. With appropriate training of raters it should be possible to achieve figures of 0.8 or 0.9 for inter-rater reliability.

Thus, by means of rating scales Dr Hart can extract from fairly dense qualitative data the exact numbers which will be entered in her data file. She has followed the same process as if coding a structured schedule but in this case the 'rules' for assignment of cases are embedded in the rating scale and in the agreement as to how it will be used. But while the logic is not dissimilar the use of rating scales has certain advantages and disadvantages over more traditional structured techniques.

Advantages

In principle the quality of the data obtained will be that much better. A structured schedule relies on one assessor, the researcher or very often patients/respondents themselves, and offers a very narrow range of options. How is one expected to answer complex questions about feeling states—such as 'Are you happy?'—in terms of 'yes/no' or 'a lot/a little' boxes? You might be happy with your job but find your golf handicap extremely worrying. Far better surely to capture an hour or so of someone talking about their life and basing rating scores on this comprehensive account. If well carried out this latter process must surely produce a more valid measure.

Structured schedules precategorize the data—a tick in a box—and if the questionnaire omitted a question it is forever lost. With unstructured data there is more flexibility for going back to the collected data to derive even more measures. Of course there is a limit to this. An in-depth interview to explore life events and mood is unlikely to be of great value in assessing eating habits, but within those constraints there may be hundreds of measures that can be derived from a couple of hours of taped interview. For example, it may be that in the assessment of self-esteem it begins to appear that the quality of the relationship with her husband is the chief determinant of a woman's own feelings of self worth; in which case it would be possible to create a rating scale for the quality of the relationship and go back to the interviews and apply it.

Disadvantages

The main disadvantage of devising rating scales to transform qualitative into quantitative data, as compared with coding structured schedules, is cost. Interviews require interviewers and, to get worthwhile material, may last an hour or more. The first ten minutes of any interview is likely to be fairly stilted, perhaps skirting around basic landmarks such as age, number of children, past illnesses, and so on, and it is only later that the important description of a respondent's more private self begins to appear. On top of the time taken to conduct the interviews is the time to devise rating scales and the time to listen again to the tapes and apply the scales. Data quality might be good, but in the time it takes to process a dozen cases it might be possible to collect and code data from several hundred structured questionnaires.

In sum, it is swings and roundabouts. You can have large amounts of rather crude data or small amounts of more sophisticated material. Which course you choose will depend very much on what your question is. Some questions are easily answered by structured questionnaires, others require the more time-consuming but finer techniques of collecting qualitative data and carefully transforming them into numbers.

QUALITATIVE METHOD

The final part of this chapter has shown how qualitative data can be transformed into numbers. The process is similar to obtaining numbers from quantitative data in that 'categories' are imposed on raw data. Arguably, the use of rating scales, as suggested above, minimizes the 'loss' of detail in the data. Even so, there is still a considerable loss and for some research the reduction of rich qualitative data to a few numbers would seem absurd. The alternative course of action is therefore to omit this stage of transformation into number entirely.

Numbers obtained from coding frames and rating scales are manipulated, generally using statistical methods, to reach a general statement about the world, such as 'Only 60 per cent of Dr Pole's patients are satisfied with his services' or 'Rheumatoid arthritics tend to have low self-esteem'. The alternative is to aim for this general statement directly from the data: there is still 'loss' of detail, but instead of abstracting numbers from the data one takes more general 'themes' and uses these as the basis of the final statement. This 'manipulation' of number and themes will be further explored in the next three chapters.

SUMMARY

This chapter has dealt with the fairly technical procedure of transforming raw data into numbers. In addition it should, on reflection, enable you to see questionnaire design and interviewing in their context: if this is your end-point, then your data collection should be so organized to enable you to get there.

SUGGESTED TASKS

1. Devise a coding frame for the therapeutic groups of your prescriptions.

    Take a sample of repeat prescriptions from your practice and code them using the above frame.

    In addition you may like to see if certain types of patients tend to receive prescriptions from certain therapeutic groups more than others. Note something of the personal characteristics of the patients receiving repeat prescriptions, code these, and compare them with your therapeutic groups. Are men more likely to get certain types of medicines compared with women? Are younger people more likely to get different types than older people?

2. Using some case notes from the practice devise a rating scale for the quality of information and legibility. Then take a random sample of case notes and, looking at the last five entries, code each using your prepared rating scale.

Are there any patterns? Do some doctors write fuller and more legible notes than others? Is it the type of illness or the type of patient that determines how good the notes are?

7   Analysing data

The previous chapter described how data were prepared and organized ready for analysis. Data come through to this stage in different forms: they can range from being fairly 'raw', perhaps in the form of qualitative data such as taped interviews or conversation transcripts, to very 'refined' in the form of a string of numbers representing the coding of responses to a questionnaire.

The analysis provides the opportunity to link the research question (from Chapter 1) directly to the data that have been collected and 'organized' (Chapter 6). The exact form of the analysis will depend on the type and quantity of data. If there are quantitative data these are likely to lead to some form of statistical exploration (discussed in Chapter 9). But there are steps to cover before this stage. Not all of these steps may be involved in any one piece of research, but by describing each in turn you should appreciate some of the basic procedures in analysing data.

WHAT SORT OF DATA DO I HAVE?

Before discussing data analysis you must be familiar with three sets of ways of categorizing data, each with its own terminology.

Is this a case, a variable, or a value?

These are terms with distinct meanings which you must be able to distinguish.

Cases
These are the individual 'things', some aspect of which is measured in research. They are most likely to be patients but they could be households, cars, tumours, or events, depending on the research question.

Variables
These are the characteristics of the cases which are measured. Patients have height, weight, blood pressure, stress, and so on, all of which are variables. Equally households have members, cars have colours and different lengths, tumours have types and sizes, and events might have seriousness and timing. For any case, it is rare to measure all the characteristics or variables it 'possesses'; it is usual only to measure those that have a bearing on the research question.

Note that depending on the research question and design the same phenomenon might be a case or a variable. For example, in an investigation of suicide attempts in a practice one might consider the patients as cases who do or do not make suicide attempts (the variable), perhaps so that the characteristics of people who make attempts (further variables) can be explored. Alternatively, the actual suicide attempts could be the cases which, in their turn, have characteristics (variables) associated with them, such as patients' names. Thus, if there are several instances of multiple attempts at suicide in the practice, the latter schema allows for each attempt to be fully described (whereas using patients as cases makes each attempt simply another characteristic of the patient).

Values

These are the 'scores' for each variable. A patient might be 1.6 metres tall, weigh 73 kilograms, have a blood pressure of 130 systolic, 80 diastolic and suffer from 1.3 units of stress on the Noddy Stress Scale. In the same way blue is the value for a car's colour, benign the value for a tumour's type, and 1945 the value for the date the Second World War ended.

EXERCISE 7.1

Are the following terms, cases, variables, or values?

1. The doctor checked Mrs Smith's *blood pressure* and found it was increased.
2. The doctor checked *Mrs Smith*'s blood pressure and found it was increased.
3. The doctor checked Mrs Smith's blood pressure and found it was *increased*.
4. *Big families* often have more illness.
5. He looked *anaemic*.
6. I checked his *haemoglobin*.
7. She has had three *heart attacks*.
8. She has had *three* heart attacks.
9. *She* has had three heart attacks.

Suggested answers can be found at the end of the chapter.

Are the variables dependent or independent?

In any research it is usual to divide the main variables into two sorts, independent and dependent. In a causal model the former is the cause, the latter the effect. Thus, in a trial of analgesics for rheumatic pain the independent variable is the analgesic while the pain is the dependent variable (both being characteristics (variables) of the patient (case) who receives the drug or experiences the pain). An independent variable is therefore the thing that produces a change in the dependent one. (You can remember it by remembering that the dependent variable is the one that 'depends' on the independent.)

In a study with many variables it is simply a question of sorting out on theoretical grounds what is supposed to affect what. A study of the effect of analgesics on rheumatic pain might also measure patients' nausea: as it is assumed that this too is brought about by the analgesic then this variable is also a dependent one. On the other hand, if the study were also to measure the patient's age, believing that this might have an effect on pain perception, then this is an independent variable.

As will be seen later, some variables are less clearly either dependent or independent. If, in the above study, it was possible to measure the placebo effect then this might be viewed as a consequence of taking the analgesic—in other words it is a dependent variable—or it might be evaluated for its effect, alongside the analgesic, on the patient's pain, and therefore be construed as an independent variable.

What is the level of measurement of the values?

Quantitative studies produce masses of numbers: but there are numbers and numbers. It is important to be aware of what numbers mean.

QUESTION 7.1

It has been suggested that different religious groups have different haemoglobin levels. To test this you conduct haemoglobin screening on one hundred of your patients and your partner does the same. The coding frame you both use for religion is as follows:

Protestant = 1
Jew   = 2
Catholic = 3
Other   = 4

Your partner reports to you that using these scores the average haemoglobin for his patients is 12.7 mg per cent and his average 'religion score' is 1.3. You have a larger Catholic population so he wonders if your average haemoglobin is different. You calculate your average haemoglobin level as 11.2 mg per cent and your religion score as 2.6—exactly twice that of your partner. 'I think it looks like the higher the religion score then the lower the haemoglobin', your partner declares. What's wrong with his conclusion?

Your partner has added together numbers which cannot be added together. Haemoglobin is measured in milligrams. We know that a milligram scale has an essential property, technically called *transitivity*. This means that one milligram is much the same as any other. Thus the 2 mg gap between 5 mg and 7 mg is exactly the same as that between 2000 mg and 2002 mg. It means that 6 mg is twice 3 mg and 9 mg is three times. The fact that the increments on a scale are each exactly the same in this way means it is an *interval scale*. Weight, length, and age are interval scales.

The 'religion scale' possesses none of these properties. The fact that Catholics were scored 3 and Protestants 1 was entirely fortuitous; it expresses no mathematical relationship but was simply a cypher or name: hence such scales are called nominal scales. Perhaps the religions could have been coded A, B, C, and D, which would have removed the temptation to add together to create an overall 'religion' score. Of course, the different haemoglobin scores (interval scales) can be added and averaged within religious groups A, B, C, and D. Thus, the correct procedure in the above study would have been to find the mean haemoglobin for each religious group, 1, 2, 3, and 4, or A, B, C, and D, and see if they were the same or, as the hypothesis suggested, different.

The third 'level of measurement' is an *ordinal scale*. As the name implies, an ordinal scale assumes some kind of underlying order or hierarchy such that it can be said that 3 is greater than 2 which in its turn is greater than 1, but it cannot be concluded that 3 is three times greater than 1 nor that 2 is twice. Imagine an interval scale of numbers in which several are randomly picked out (the ones in bold type):

$$1 \ \mathbf{2} \ 3 \ 4 \ \mathbf{5} \ \mathbf{6} \ 7 \ 8 \ \mathbf{9} \ 10 \ 11 \ 12 \ \mathbf{13} \ \mathbf{14} \ 15$$

These numbers, 2, 5, 6, 9, 13, 14, are parts of an interval scale (6 is three times 2), but they could be transposed into an ordinal scale by numbering the first number 1, the second 2, the third 3, and so on. The result is the following scale (with the original numbers in parentheses)

$$1(2) \ 2(5) \ 3(6) \ 4(9) \ 5(13) \ 6(14)$$

You can see now that though the new scale looks like an interval one—running from 1 to 6—the numbers do not have the same properties as those in an interval scale. Thus, in this ordinal scale it is certain that 2 is not twice 1 (in fact it is two and a half times). In ordinal scales, the size of the 'gap' between the numbers is not known (otherwise it could be expressed as an interval scale), all that can be said is that 2 is larger than 1 and 3 is larger than 1 and 2, and so on—but this is quite a lot more than can be said about a nominal scale.

Take, for example, a study to examine prescribing practices amongst different doctors. Say there is to be a comparison between house officers, registrars, and consultants. Coding each grade of doctor respectively 1, 2, and 3, it might reasonably be claimed that this is an ordinal scale. It certainly is not interval—two house officers do not make the exact equivalent of a registrar—but neither is it nominal, because there is an order or hierarchy to the scale: a consultant is 'more' in the sense of experience or qualifications than a registrar who in turn is more than a house officer.

At this stage it might appear a bit like an academic game trying to decide the level of measurement employed, but knowing this is important, as will be seen, both in understanding what the data mean and in choosing an appropriate statistical test.

EXERCISE 7.2

Examine the following questionnaire and assess each question as either using nominal, ordinal, or interval scales.

Patient questionnaire

1. What is your age in years?
2. Are you male or female   male ❏

            female ❏
3. What is your occupation?
4. How long have you been registered
  with your GP?

        0–5 years ❏

        6–10 years ❏

     11 or more years ❏
5. Would you describe your health as:

        very good ❏

          good ❏

          poor ❏

        very poor ❏
6. Have you ever forgotten to take your tablets
  for your high blood pressure? yes ❏

            no ❏
7. Mark somewhere on the line below your level
  of satisfaction with your treatment.

very satisfied   middling   very dissatisfied

 |--| --------------------------------------|

       Suggested answers can be found at the end of the chapter.

DATA CHECKING

It goes without saying that the accuracy of the underlying data is important in any analysis. The whole research process up to this point has been designed to ensure that the data are 'valid', but in addition it is necessary to ensure that there are no silly errors from miscoding and mispunching. This requires checking the coding and, if resources permit, double-punching the data. There are, in addition, a couple of useful initial procedures with which to start the exploration of the data: these are in fact part of the analysis but they might also identify any errors that have been made earlier.

First, it is customary to check *frequencies*. This means, in simple terms, seeing how 'frequently' various values occur. (This process is described in the next chapter using the Epi Info software program.) Thus, if a study measured the smoking habits of a practice population it is useful just to do simple additions. What is the frequency of smokers in the adult population? 30 per cent? 40 per cent? This is what might be expected from national studies; if it turns out that there are only 10 per cent or perhaps as many as 90 per cent then before proceeding it is worth checking the figures: either there is a mistake somewhere, or there is a very unusual population, or there might be a discovery of some interest.

Similarly, if a study involved measuring consultation rates per patient it would be useful to know the mean (average) for the practice together with the range. The national average is around 3 or 4 per year. About 20 per cent of patients do not consult in any one year (so we expect a good proportion of 0s in the data) and some consult quite frequently. But if it is found that someone seems to have consulted 80 times last year it probably bears checking out: it may be correct but it is more likely to be an error than a figure of 4 consultations per year would be.

More obviously, the frequencies check will clearly show up 'illegal values'. Thus, in a study of the proportions of men and women amongst doctor-initiated consultations it is likely that males and females would be coded as 1 and 2, respectively. However, if the frequencies show a number of 3s then it would suggest that either there has been a miscoding on the original questionnaire, or the data have been mispunched into the data file. A check with the original questionnaires (using the patient's code number as an identifier) will quickly show the error.

In summary, by checking on outlying and illegal values the researcher will have more confidence in the accuracy of the data set. Moreover, this process has the added bonus of increasing familiarity with the distribution of values in the data. For example, in a study of the relationship between housing tenure and consultations for URTIs, the relative absence of owner-occupiers might already begin to suggest interesting hypotheses.

The second way you might be able to check your data is by looking for *internal consistency*. Are all your examples of gynaecological problems to be found in women? A miscoded man would clearly stand out. Are all the people for whom you have details of number of cigarettes smoked also scored as smokers? It is possible to fail to get details of numbers of cigarettes smoked from someone scored as a smoker, but if a ten-a-day patient is also coded as a non-smoker then something is wrong somewhere.

At the end of this preliminary analysis you will have:

- completed another check on the data
- some basic descriptive statistics of the data
- even more familiarity with the data which should stand in good stead when exploring it further.

HANDLING NON-RESPONDERS

Almost all data collection produces blanks: patients who refused, notes that were missing, data that was illegible, and so on. One of the earliest parts of an analysis is to look at this 'non-response'.

The main question to be answered is: are the non-responders different from the responders? If they are not different, then it can fairly be assumed that had they responded (or had the notes not been lost, or whatever) then they would have answered in a similar way to responders. The way to check this, as advised earlier, is to collect whatever data are available on non-responders so they can be compared.

Say, in a survey of symptom experience, 30 per cent of the sample refuse to complete the questionnaire. If you manage to collect at least the age and sex of each of these non-responders then it is possible to see if their age and sex distribution mirrors that of the responders. If it does, then you can assume that their symptom experience would be likely to mirror that of the sample too. Of course, the more data available with which to make comparisons between responders and non-responders then the more confidently the sameness (or difference) of the two groups can be assumed. If the non-responders seem to be similar to the responders then analysis of the data can proceed with some confidence that the responders are not atypical.

But what if the non-responders are significantly different in some way? Does this jeopardize the whole research study? Well, it does mean that conclusions must be that much more tentative, though it may be possible to allow for some of the bias. For example, if you were to find that the non-responders were similar to the responders except they tended to be older then it would seem wise, when analysing the responders, to pay particular attention to age as a variable. Thus, if it was found that older people tend to report more symptoms then, in light of the relative excess of elderly in the 'missing' part of the sample, it is probable that the population experiences more symptoms overall than the data from the responders might indicate. And with the number of 'missing' elderly known it may even be possible to estimate (from the responses of elderly people included in the responders) what symptoms they would have reported.

TWO-VARIABLE TABLES

There are now many complex statistical procedures that enable several variables to be analysed together—so-called 'multivariate' techniques. At some stage you may wish to master these techniques, but be warned that despite the appeal of an analysis that promises to show the interrelationships between all the variables at once there is often difficulty in interpreting the result. Even after a virtuoso performance with multivariate statistics, researchers often come back to the basic building blocks of analysis: the relationship between two or three variables. This is as much as this chapter will cover, as these are the most useful analytic tools. Let us start with two variables.

Unless a study is a simple descriptive one, for example 'How many asthmatics consult every year?', two or more variables will have been measured for each case in the sample. Let us imagine you are interested in whether your female patients consult more frequently than male ones. The cases are the patients. For each case, two variables are measured, namely patient's sex and number of consultations in a certain time period. For each variable in each case there is a value, male or female, and a number between, say, 0 and 10.

We can now draw up a 'table' which would look like this:

Consultations in year

		0 1 2 3 4 5 6 7 8 9 10
Sex	Male	
	Female	

We can then assign each case to a 'cell' in the table. If the first case in the sample, a Mr Aaron, did not consult in the year under consideration then he goes into the top left cell; the second case, Mrs Bell, who consulted three times would go into the bottom row, fourth cell along; and so on. The result might be something like what we see in Table 7.1. This is a rather cumbersome table with 20 cells, many of which are empty. It can therefore be helpful to 'collapse down' the stretched out 'interval' scale into a shorter ordinal one. Let's divide the group between 'high' consulters having four or more consultations per year and 'low' consulters having three or less. Table 7.2 is the redrawn version.

Table 7.1 *Consultations in year*

		0	1	2	3	4	5	6	7	8	9	10
Sex	Male	10	16	20	10	6	3	0	0	1	0	0
	Female	2	1	4	3	1	2	1	0	0	0	1

Table 7.2 *Consulters*

		Low	High	Totals
Sex	Male	56	10	66
	Female	10	5	15

At first sight it might appear that men are over 2 times more likely to be high consulters than women from this data (10 versus 5 cases respectively). However, this conclusion is mistaken because there are different sized groups of men and women—somehow the sample managed to include far more men than women (66 against 15). The question being asked is not 'What is the most likely gender of my next patient?'—which, from these figures would be male—but 'Comparing any individual man or woman, who is more likely to be a high consulter?' The

Table 7.3 *Consulters*

		Low	High	
Sex	Male	85	15	100%
	Female	67	33	100%

Table 7.4 *Consulters*

		Low	High
Sex	Male	85	67
	Female	15	33
		100%	100%

way to answer this question is to express the results as percentages. Thus we can compile Table 7.3.

It now looks fairly clear that women tend to be higher consulters then men: fully one third of women are high consulters in this table compared with only 15 per cent of men. This could be explored further by carrying out relevant statistical tests on either this table (or the first full one, Table 7.1) to see whether this distribution of consultation rates might have occurred by chance.

A NOTE ON PERCENTAGING

In Table 7.3, percentages were calculated across the rows, ensuring that the figure 100 per cent summed either all the men or all the women. The percentaging could, of course, also have been calculated down the columns, making the 100 per cent figure cover either low or high consulters. Deriving such a table from the original numbers in Table 7.2 gives us Table 7.4. From this table it is tempting to draw the opposite conclusion than from Table 7.3: whereas in the latter table women seemed to be twice as likely to be high consulters as men, in this table—based on exactly the same data—it is the men who seem to be twice as likely to be high consulters than women. Which interpretation is correct? In terms of the original question, Table 7.3 is correct. It is possible to use Table 7.4 but it answers a different sort of question. The usual rule to follow is to make the independent variable total 100 per cent in the table's margins because it is the effect of the independent variable on the dependent one, in this case the effect of gender on consultation rates, that is important.

Table 7.5

		X		
		Present	Absent	
Y	Present			
	Absent			

Table 7.6

		X		
		Present	Absent	
Y	Present	100	0	100%
	Absent	0	100	100%

Papers do get published in which the researchers have percentaged in the wrong direction, so be on the look out for this mistake. Incidentally, it makes no difference whether the independent variable is placed along the top or down the side of the table so long as the percentage is calculated in the right direction (across or down respectively).

THREE-VARIABLE ANALYSIS

For simple questions, analysis can stop at the two-variable stage. But the apparent relationship—or lack of one—between two variables can be further explored by adding in a third.

The logic behind this is simple. If there are two variables, X and Y, which are assigned values, say, present or absent, a 2×2 table can be constructed (as shown above for gender and consultation rates) as in Table 7.5.

It is possible, though very unlikely in any research study, to have data which shows a perfect relationship between X and Y such than when X is present Y is present and when X is absent Y is absent. See Table 7.6, for example.

Much more likely is to have relationships which suggest that Y is *partly* explained by X, as in Table 7.7. What this table means is that X certainly has an effect on Y, in fact quite a strong one, but change in Y is also being affected by some other factors; what causes Y to be present in the absence of X (top right-hand corner) and why does X have no effect on Y in over a quarter of all instances (bottom left-hand corner)? It is virtually impossible that your research is going to identify all the factors which affect Y such that change in Y is perfectly explained,

Table 7.7

		X Present	Absent	
Y	Present	80	20	100%
	Absent	27	73	100%

Table 7.8

		Attenders	Control
MI	Yes	5	2
	No	95	98
		100%	100%

but you can get further than Table 7.7 by introducing other variables which might influence Y, and look for their effect.

SPECIFICATION

The process of examining the effect of introducing a third variable into an existing relationship between two variables is often called *elaboration* or *specification* because it is trying to elaborate or specify the form of the relationship between the first two variables. There are many ways a third variable might affect another two. Two hypothetical examples follow that give a flavour of what can be found.

Example 1: The case of the iatrogenic clinic

For several years a practice ran a health promotion clinic for interested patients. It was then decided to evaluate the service, and those men who had attended the clinic were compared with a control group of men of similar background who had not attended. By examining the notes, all myocardial infarctions in both groups were recorded. The partners were horrified to discover that the highest rate of infarcts (in fact twice as many) was in the group who had attended the clinic (see Table 7.8). The original hypothesis, that attendance at the clinic would benefit the patients, seemed to have been challenged (ignoring for the moment the fact that only very small numbers are involved).

However, there are other possible explanations for this finding: the most promising is to argue that people who attended the clinic were more likely to be at risk in the first place, through either a poor family history or early signs of ischaemic heart disease, and this had induced them to try the clinic. Fortunately

Table 7.9 *Patients with a history of heart diseas*

		Attenders	Control
MI	Yes	5 (9%)	1 (10%)
	No	55 (91%)	9 (90%)
		100%	100%

Table 7.10 *Patients without a history of heart disease*

		Attenders	Control
MI	Yes	0 (0%)	1 (1%)
	No	40 (100%)	89 (99%)
		100%	100%

the GPs had recorded the patients' previous histories, so it was possible to intro-duce them as a third variable into the analysis. In Table 7.9 only those men with any previous history of heart problems are included; in Table 7.10 only those without such a history. In effect, a previous history is being 'controlled out'.

From these tables it is possible to see that the clinic, in fact, was not doing damage. Rather than the apparent model:

clinic attendance   →   ischaemic heart disease

it seems that the better model is:

previous history   →   ischaemic heart disease
            ↘
                  clinic attendance

in which a history of heart disease caused both attendance and the increased likelihood of an actual infarct.

Example 2: The case of the negative result

Concerned that unemployment might be causing ill health, a GP recorded the consultation rate of 100 of her patients who were unemployed and 100 employed patients to act as controls. She divided the consultation rates into two groups, low and high consulters. Placing the results into a table she found no difference between the two groups of patients: see Table 7.11.

Table 7.11 *All patients*

		Employed	Unemployed
Consultations	High	15	15
	Low	85	85
		100%	100%

Table 7.12 *Young patients*

		Employed	Unemployed
Consultations	High	1 (2%)	12 (50%)
	Low	59 (98%)	13 (50%)
		100%	100%

Table 7.13 *Old patients*

		Employed	Unemployed
Consultations	High	14 (35%)	3 (4%)
	Low	26 (65%)	72 (96%)
		100%	100%

Perplexed at this finding, the GP decided to examine the relationship between employment and consulting, controlling for other factors. First she tried age, dividing the group into those under and over 40 (young/old). She obtained the data shown in Tables 7.12 and 7.13. From these it would appear that there was in fact a relationship between unemployment and consulting behaviour: for young men it increased, but for older men it was diminished. The original Table 7.11 had combined both influences and effectively cancelled out these two findings. It now would be interesting to go on and control for gender, as it might be hypothesized that men would react worse than women to unemployment; and then with other variables.

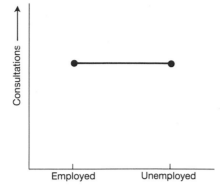

Figure 7.1 Diagram showing relationship of employment to consultations.

A NOTE ON PRESENTATION

Both the above examples used tables to present the data. After these have been put together it takes a few minutes' study to decide what exactly they are showing. The quickest way of seeing whether a 2×2 table contains anything of positive significance is to do a rough multiplication of the numbers at the end of the two diagonals: if they are roughly the same then the two variables in the table have little or no influence on each other; if, on the other hand, there is a large difference in the two sums obtained then there must be a large effect of one variable on the other.

There are alternatives to tables: for early exploration of the data, graphs or histograms can be very useful. For example, when the dependent variable takes the form of an interval or ordinal scale, as in the last example, it is possible to get a visual comparison of the effect of two and three variables.

First let us see Table 7.11 plotted on a graph (but using the actual consultation scale rather than the reduced two-value scale).

The line in Fig. 7.1 shows the relationship between the two variables: it is flat because both employed and unemployed have the same 'rate' on the left-hand scale. Now introduce the third variable, age. This can be represented by two lines, one for younger and one for older men. It is now clear from Fig. 7.2 that for each age group employment status does have an effect on consultations as shown by the slope to the line; moreover, because the slopes are in opposite directions it can be concluded, as above, that the form of the relationship between employment and consultation varies inversely with age.

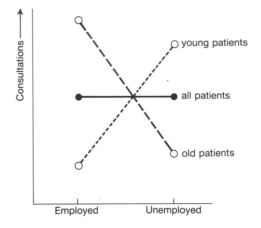

Figure 7.2 Diagram showing relationship of employment and age to consultations.

MANIPULATING VARIABLES

Earlier, it was shown how people above and below a certain age could be aggregated into two age groups. In effect, the age variable was 'collapsed' so reducing the possible values the variable 'age' could possess from a hundred or so to two (young/old) or at least many fewer (0–9, 10–19, 20–29, and so on). In the same way, existing variables can be manipulated to create new ones. Let us look at three ways of creating new variables.

Rates

One of the most useful new variables to calculate is a rate. For example, if you have been comparing prescribing amongst the partners in your practice you may have first measured how many prescriptions everyone wrote last week:

	Number of prescriptions
Doctor A	80
Doctor B	40
Doctor C	50

Doctor A clearly wrote the most, fully twice as many as Doctor B. If you felt the practice was writing too many prescriptions Doctor A would seem a good person to start with. Or would he? Another way of looking at the results is to calculate a rate which would express the number of prescriptions as a proportion of some relevant denominator. In this instance the denominator might be the

Table 7.14

	Number of patients' prescriptions	Number of patients	Rate per 100 patients
Doctor A	80	160	50
Doctor B	40	120	33
Doctor C	50	90	56

number of patients seen last week (and then multiplied by 100 to get a prescription rate per 100 patients). This achieves the result shown in Table 7.14. The picture now looks quite different. The highest prescriber is not Doctor A but Doctor C.

There are of course other denominators which could have been used, such as personal list size, or the length of surgeries. In each case a choice must be made as to the most appropriate for the question in hand, but in each case this new variable can be used in the analyses in place of the 'raw' prescription numbers.

More complex combinations

In studies of risk factors, obesity may well be important. The commonest way of operationalizing obesity is by measuring weight. However, a weight that makes one person obese might be normal in someone much taller. The solution has been to combine height and weight in a new variable using the formula

$$\frac{weight}{height^2} = \text{Body Mass Index}$$

From starting with two variables there are now three: two have been combined (or reduced, as it is often described) into an index. All three variables can be used in further analyses, but it is much more common to continue only with the new one which is superior in certain ways to the old ones.

Indices

The process of reducing variables to a summary index is a common one. In the above example it was achieved by multiplication and division, but it is often carried out simply by addition.

Say you are interested in patient satisfaction. You design a questionnaire to measure it, asking about satisfaction with the doctor's manner, competence, and facilities. If each of these areas was scored out of five then it would be possible to create a new 'general' variable of satisfaction by adding a patient's score on each of these 'sub-dimensions' of satisfaction, in effect producing a new index or scale running from 0 to 15 which can then be related to other variables that were measured.

This is the principle of index creation and is the basis of many measures in common use. An IQ score, for example, is a summation of different test items corrected for age; a personality test usually involves summing the results of a lot of different items; the General Health Questionnaire—a common psychiatric screening instrument—produces a single score by adding together questionnaire items. You can look at a diagnosis as a sort of index because various items (signs, symptoms, and investigations) have gone together to create a new overall summary category.

Chapter 3 described how concepts were operationalized. For some, such as age, it was easy; for others, such as 'the quality of a relationship', it was more difficult, requiring a series of different questions to tap different components or dimensions of the concept. Now, at the analysis stage, it is sometimes possible to put the components together again and create the variable that could not be measured directly.

A word of caution, however. Creating an index or new variable might seem like an easy task but there are difficulties which can make it very tricky. For example, taking the supposed three dimensions of patient satisfaction mentioned above: satisfaction with doctor's manner, competence, and facilities. If, as suggested, these were added then it makes the following assumptions.

• The three five-point scales on which patients scored their satisfaction were in fact interval scales and not just ordinal (otherwise they could not legitimately be added together).
• Each of the three 'dimensions' has equal importance or weight otherwise one of the scales could have been 'weighted' (perhaps taking double the values of one which seemed 'doubly' important) in the calculation of the overall index.

In practice these two problems can make index construction a rather difficult business, especially when many variables are involved. There are some techniques available to help, but usually various assumptions have to be made. In terms of your own research, do try 'data reduction' by creating a new index out of small numbers of original variables but remember to treat any results cautiously. New variables can be used in the analysis like the original ones, just as above.

QUALITATIVE DATA AND ANALYSIS

The 'rules' for analysing qualitative data are less precise than for quantitative data. In quantitative data the search is for patterns between variables using devices such as two- and three-variable tables to bring these to attention. For qualitative data there is no such easy mechanism, though the same basic goal guides the analysis.

Look for variables or themes

In qualitative, as for quantitative, research there are cases and for each case some data. But it is not at first clear what the variables are, because these emerge from the analysis. For example, in studying patient satisfaction a questionnaire captures the researcher's views of what are important variables. The patient simply has to assign these variables particular values—a lot, not much, a little, and so on. A qualitative approach to researching satisfaction, on the other hand, would perhaps invite patients to talk about how they saw satisfaction in general. The analysis then consists of looking at all the transcripts and drawing out the sorts of things that have concerned patients—which might be quite different from the ones the researcher might have imagined would be of concern. These patient-defined concerns are in effect the study variables.

Identify more general statements or hypotheses which link variables

In the analysis of quantitative data it is usual to look at the values assigned to each variable of each case so as to explore the relationship between them. In a qualitative study it might not be necessary to go to the specific values before picking out a relationship between two or more variables. A patient who complains about surgery times because he works long hours allows the generation of a hypothesis that work patterns might affect patients' evaluations of surgery opening times. Then go on to other cases to see if a similar pattern emerges elsewhere. This process might be seen as equivalent to exploring the relationship between two variables in a table.

Then, akin to adding other variables, look for other patterns of relationships between work hours and surgery convenience: is it only men who complain about this? Is it evening and morning surgeries which are criticized? And so on. The end-result is a statement which somehow captures what are the relationships hidden in the data.

QUANTITATIVE AND QUALITATIVE ANALYSIS COMPARED

It might appear that a quantitative demonstration of the relationship between working hours and practice facilities would be better than a qualitative one. Several points can be made in response:

• A quantitative study might not have measured these variables, not believing any of them to be important (though it would be possible to do so now that their importance has been suggested).

• A quantitative study tends to capture a response in a formal box; respondents might give a more valid answer if allowed freely to express their ideas in their own words. The quality of data thus tends to be better.

• Sometimes 'patterns' in data that might be missed in a quantitative analysis can be more easily seen in qualitative data.

Taken together these points suggest that analysis of qualitative data, for all its seeming lack of precision, may produce important and interesting conclusions which would have been missed using more conventional techniques.

THE RESEARCH QUESTION IN THE CONTEXT OF THEORY

In Chapter 1 the importance of starting research with a question was stressed. That advice still stands, but now can be put into a context. A research question ('What is the relationship between variable X and variable Y?') is not an isolated statement, but belongs to a group of lots of other statements about X and about Y. The single two-variable question is simply one component in a network of many interconnected variables that together make up 'theory'. For example, the statement that stress causes heart attacks is just one linkage out of all the other factors that cause or influence in some way both heart attacks and stress.

In a rather simple way the outline of a theory began to emerge above in the hypothetical exploration of the relationship between attendance at a health promotion clinic, a history of heart disease, and myocardial infarction. Introducing more variables into that relationship would have allowed further progress in understanding the role of all the factors involved.

The important message is that while the original research question might only involve two variables it would be foolish just to measure and analyse those two variables alone. As was shown above, no relationship between two variables might be shown until other variables were introduced. Therefore in any research project it is important to try to tap and measure other variables that might have an influence, even though they do not necessarily occur explicitly in the original research question.

How do you choose what to measure? In part this comes from the theoretical context of the question being asked. If you are carrying out a study of a supposed aetiological factor for ischaemic heart disease then it would seem wise to include known risk factors, such as smoking, in the measurement process. Then there are some variables that on the basis of previous studies are known to have very general effects; it would be valuable to include them even though there might be no known connection between them and your question variables. Some socio-demographic variables, such as age and sex, seem worth measuring in any study of patients simply because they are so frequently found to relate to other variables.

In qualitative research, there is less choice of what variables to include in the study as what is seen and heard 'in the field' is the more important guide. Thus, an observational study of a surgery waiting room will be dependent to a large extent on what actually happens there while it is being observed; or an interview with a patient on chronic illness will depend on what the patient has to say. Nevertheless, there is still need for guidance—what to look for, what prompts to give the patient—and these too will depend on having thought through the wider context of the research question in hand.

FINGERS, SLIDE RULES, AND COMPUTERS

Theory is important in another aspect of analysis. Nowadays most analysis is carried out by computer. The sorts of tables constructed and discussed above can be called up almost instantly on a computer. Because of this there is a temptation to ask the computer for all possible tables in a sort of fishing trip for 'significant' results. However, this is not a substitute for properly thinking through the meaning and interpretation of the data. As described above, two variables can be explored in one table; however, examination of all the paired relationships between three variables will take three tables; and four variables will take six; five will take ten; and so on. Add in the tables generated by controlling for a third variable and very rapidly there might be several hundred tables if the computer is asked to trawl every possible relationship. In addition to constructing the table the computer can also give an instant evaluation of whether a particular relationship is statistically 'significant'. An advantage? Well yes, except that using standard 'levels' of significance one in twenty tables will be reported as 'significant' simply by chance—and there is no way of discriminating these from 'really' significant results.

Use computers for analysis by all means, they are a great boon. There are now many statistical 'packages' available which will help you with the analyses outlined above; some of these packages work on personal computers so if you have a PC in the practice you might well be able to do the analysis on it (see the next chapter on using one such software program). It will make the statistical tests covered in Chapter 9 very easy. However, do not be seduced into believing that computers will do your thinking for you. It's your question, they are your data, do not let the computer take them over. The logic of analysis, as this module suggests, can be pursued quite independently of machines.

SUMMARY

This module has described the types of data produced from a research project and the way to go about starting to analyse it using two- and three-variable tables. These tables will suggest interesting relationships between variables. The generation of these tables using a PC is described in the next chapter; Chapter 9 discusses the selection of appropriate statistical tests.

SUGGESTED TASKS

Monitor one week's surgeries, noting the age of each patient and whether they get a prescription or not. Draw up 2 × 2 tables to show the results. You would do this by splitting the ages into two groups; see the effects of splitting at different ages, such as greater or less than 40, greater or less than 65, and so on.

ANSWERS TO EXERCISES

EXERCISE 7.1

1. *Blood pressure* is a variable
2. *Mrs Smith* is a case
3. *increased* is a value
4. *Big families* are cases
5. *anaemic* is a value
6. *haemoglobin* is a variable (of which anaemia is a value)
7. *heart attacks* are either case or variable depending on study design: is it patients or heart attacks which are being studied?
8. *three* is a value (of heart attacks)
9. *she* is a case.

EXERCISE 7.2

1. age: interval ratio scale
2. sex: nominal scale
3. occupation: nominal scale—though if it were transformed into social class it would become an ordinal one
4. time registered: interval ratio scale
5. health: ordinal scale
6. compliance: nominal scale
7. satisfaction: ordinal scale. (A visual analogue scale such as this might appear like an interval scale because exact gaps between responses can be measured. However, it is known that respondents are more inclined to mark a point towards the centre and ignore the extremes: this suggests that every millimetre of the scale does not have the same meaning for the respondent.)

8 Using data analysis software

Data analysis can be carried out manually, but the availability of personal computers (PCs) makes the task much easier and allows a more rigorous examination of the data. There are a number of different data analysis packages available in the market, and, to confuse the computer illiterate, a number of different computer standards. This chapter is about using a particular data analysis package with an IBM-compatible PC: if you do not have access to this kind of computer then you should skip the latter part of the chapter. However, for all interested readers, here is a brief overview of computers and software.

PERSONAL COMPUTERS

It was the advent of the microprocessor about 20 years ago that allowed the emergence of desktop computers. Previously, computers had occupied whole rooms and were strictly for the very technically minded. The potential of these new machines was slowly realized as a number of different types emerged to cater for games enthusiasts, business, and various specialist applications. And as the uses for the machines expanded, the underlying technology increased in leaps and bounds so that today's desktop computer has a capacity far in excess of most 'big' computers from the pre-microprocessor days—and costs a fraction of the price.

A number of manufacturers targeted their computers at games enthusiasts: such machines are still available (such as the Amiga and Atari computers) together with those computers which have dispensed with a keyboard so as not to distract from the game (the best known being Nintendo and Sega). In an attempt to widen the appeal of games computers some work-related programmes (such as wordprocessors) have been produced, but on balance such machines are not really suitable for serious work as the support for this side of their capability is very limited.

Serious computer users turn to two distinct types of desktop computer, the Macintosh and the IBM PC. They differ in terms of their internal structure (their hardware) and their operating systems. The latter is the basic program that allows the user and any applications (software), such as a wordprocessor, to communicate with the hardware. The Mac and its accompanying operating system is sold exclusively by Apple: this has enabled the manufacturer to control tightly the relationship between the computer and the user. The result is an operating system that is particularly easy to use: the boast is that anyone can operate a Mac in five minutes. It also means that all software whether it is a wordprocessor, database, or game, has a similar 'feel' to the user.

IBM, the big computer manufacturer, produced a rival machine—the so-called IBM PC. This uses an operating system called MS-DOS, produced by a separate software company. An important decision was to make the PC expandable and soon other manufacturers started producing add-on bits. Very quickly IBM lost control of its creation. Clone makers started buying-in the different parts and producing their own machines—hence the new generic standard of an 'IBM-compatible' computer. These clones now completely dominate the market, and indeed the PC is now of such modular construction that it is possible to buy the parts separately and put them together at home.

The benefit to consumers of this competition has been enormous. While the power of PCs increases, the price has consistently fallen; this has meant that the PC has become by far the most popular computer standard. In its turn this has meant that software producers have had more of an incentive to become involved in the PC market than the Mac. The net result is that PCs have tended to be cheaper than Macs and have a much greater choice of software available. The Mac still has its easy-to-use operating system but even this is being rivalled by the Windows interface on PCs in recent years.

THE OPERATING SYSTEM

A computer works by interpreting streams of binary numbers such as 011100100110. It is clearly impractical to type these in all the time, so the computer is provided with an operating system enabling certain words or letters to call up the appropriate stream of binary numbers. The operating system is, in effect, the interface between the hardware and you, the user. All IBM-compatible PCs use an operating system called DOS (MS-DOS or the rival Novell DR-DOS).

Many practice-based systems use an operating system based on Unix, a system usually found on larger computers. If you have such a system you will be unable to run software intended to run under MS-DOS on PCs. On the other hand, if your system uses MS-DOS then you can add standard MS-DOS software (including Epi Info, as described later) subject to your contract with the system's vendor.

SOFTWARE

There are a number of data analysis or statistical packages on the market. Perhaps the most commonly used is SPSS/PC (Statistical Package for the Social Sciences-PC version). It is a very sophisticated program and can be recommended (both authors use it), but it needs time to learn to use and is expensive. Universities often have site licences to use it, so you may be able to contact your local department of general practice to see if they can demonstrate it for you, and perhaps allow you to analyse your data on one of their computers. But there are alternatives.

Many spreadsheets have quite sophisticated data manipulation facilities as well as some basic statistical functions. The same goes for databases: with a little ingenuity, they will allow you to analyse a data set. If you already use a spreadsheet or database you might want to consider this route, but it is probably not worth buying and learning how to use such a program just to analyse your research data, especially as there is a much easier and cheaper solution.

EPI INFO

In an attempt to provide a data analysis package that would be suitable for investigating disease outbreaks in less developed countries, the World Health Organization got together with the Centres for Disease Control in Atlanta, Georgia, to produce a program called Epi Info. While intended for epidemiological surveillance, the core of the program is a data analysis module that can easily be adapted for general practice research. Moreover, the program has been placed in the public domain—which means that it is free and its distribution is encouraged.

The program has been written to work under MS-DOS on PCs. The program itself comes on a standard single high density 3½-inch disk so your computer will need a drive that can read such disks. (It is possible to get the program on two medium density 3½-inch disks or even on four 5¼-inch disks, but you will have to persuade someone to do this for you.) You will need to copy the program from the floppy disk (it is stored in compressed files) on to a hard disk. The full program occupies about 2 megabytes of space on the hard disk but if certain files are omitted—which have more relevance to epidemiologists—it only needs just over 1.5 megabytes of space.

You should be able to get a copy of Epi Info from the Public Health Department of your local health authority, or from your local academic department of general practice for little more than the cost of a blank disk and a postage stamp.

Installing Epi Info on your hard disk

Note

- <RTN> indicates that you should press the 'return' or 'enter' key
- commands you should type into your computer are given in italics.

Epi Info is installed by placing the floppy (or first floppy of the series) in the floppy drive and changing the DOS prompt to that drive. (You should consult your DOS manual if you are unclear as to how to do this.)

Type *install* <RTN>. The programme prompts you to say which drive you are reading the disk from, and the drive to which you wish to send the files. There are two options here. One is to send the files to another floppy for copying for another person. (This copying facility also enables you to transfer the files from 3½-inch to 5¼-inch disks and to and from low and high density disks.) The other option is to install the program files on to your hard disk and this requires you to enter the letter indicating the hard drive you wish to install on to. The program itself then creates a sub-directory called EPI5 and proceeds to install the relevant files.

You will be prompted to say which groups of files you wish to install. If you have the space on your hard disk the easiest is to install all the files. However, if you are constrained for space the minimum to install are Groups 1 to 4 and Group 9.

At the end of the installation the program offers you the option of changing your AUTOEXEC.BAT file so that the EPI5 sub-directory is in your path. Put simply, this means that you can access Epi Info from any sub-directory without having to enter the EPI5 sub-directory specifically. If you accept this option you can then type *epi* <RTN> to enter the program. Otherwise you need to ensure that you are in the right sub-directory first by typing *cd\epi5* <RTN>.

The title screen

The title screen shows a list of programs on the left-hand side; you can move down the list using the cursor keys. On the right-hand side a brief description of the contents of each program is shown. The three programs that are of immediate interest are EPED, ENTER, and ANALYSIS. These programs enable you to go through the three basic steps of data analysis. These involve:

• creating a template of your data using the editor EPED
• entering your data into the template using ENTER
• analysing the resulting data file using ANALYSIS.

Creating a template

Enter the text editor, EPED, by placing the cursor on the program name and <RTN>. You will then be put into the editor which is made up of a blank screen with a list of function keys along the top. At any time you can press function key F1 to obtain help on the various options open to you. The help is context sensitive, that is if you press F7 then F1 it will offer advice on the F7 key. The <ESC> escape key always takes you back to your earlier point.

EPED is a basic wordprocessor and can be used for writing letters, reports, etc. However, for your present purposes you will need its ability to write a template of your data collection schedule. To write a template the only setting you need to check is that the wordwrap (which means that at the end of a line the next word moves automatically to the next line) is set to 'off'. To do this press F6 to obtain a list of setup features, place the cursor on WW (for wordwrap) and <RTN>. You will then see a sub-menu with the words 'Wordwrap ON/OFF'. The ON/OFF is toggled by pressing <RTN>. This means that when it says `OFF it can be changed to ON by pressing <RTN> and vice versa. Ensure that OFF is on the screen and press the escape key twice to return to the main screen.

Epi Info uses the term 'questionnaire' to embrace any data collection schedule. Thus, you might produce a questionnaire to give to patients (you could do it using the wordprocessing facility of EPED) but then you will need to design an abbreviated version of that questionnaire as a template for data entry. Similarly, if you have used an extraction schedule to take clinical data from the case notes you will also need to design a separate template.

Dr Abi Ofni has just completed a survey of the diabetes care in her practice. She designed a data extraction schedule on her wordprocessor. It looked like this:

Diabetes survey
1 Patient's survey number?
2 Patient's age?
3 Patient's sex?
4 What is the value of the last random blood glucose?
5 Were feet inspected in last year?

She is now ready to create her template in EPED. You should find it useful to follow her work on your own computer. First she types a heading *Diabetes Survey* in the top left corner and presses <RTN> twice. (The title could be under-lined by using the text key F4 and choosing 'Style of Type', but for the moment she decides to keep to simple text). Next she types *Number*, followed by three spaces, and then two hash symbols (##). (Depending on how your keyboard is set up these may be available as keys or they can be found by holding down the <ALT> key and pressing the numbers 3 followed by 5 on the numeric keyboard, then releasing the <ALT> key.) Alternatively, she could have obtained the hash symbols by pressing F4, placing the cursor on 'Questions', <RTN>, and then putting the cursor on the 'hash' symbols and <RTN> again. The prompt asks for how many digits before and after the decimal point and places the appropriate number of hash marks on the screen.

The hash symbols mark the places where digits will later be entered into the template. Their exact number is therefore important. Dr Ofni has 35 patients in her survey so she will require space for two digits (to range from 01 to 35). If she had over 100 patients then she would have needed three hash symbols for the three digits.

Next, she presses <RTN> to move to the next line. She types *Age*, then three spaces, and then two hash symbols (##). Then to the next line and *Sex*, three spaces, and one #. She presses <RTN> twice and types *Blood glucose*, two spaces, then ##.#. And finally on the next line she types *Feet inspected*, three spaces, then one #. Her template is now complete and looks like this:

Diabetes Survey

Number ##
Age   ##

Sex #

Blood glucose ##.#
Feet inspected #

The template bears a very close resemblance to her schedule. Indeed, she could have saved her schedule as an unformatted ASCII file on her wordprocessor and then read it into EPED (using the F2 key and choosing to open file). Then all she has to do is add the necessary hash symbols to each question. The disadvantage with this method is that Epi Info chooses the variable names (that will be used in the analysis) from the text preceding the hash symbol. Although Epi Info will recognize question numbers and will ignore certain words such as 'a' and 'the' as well as spaces, the resulting variable name can be cumbersome. Thus, while reducing 'Blood sugar' to a variable BLOODSUGAR (maximum of ten letters), it would reduce '4 What is the value of the last random blood glucose?' to N4WHATISVA. The former more clearly indicates the nature of this particular variable. Even so, Dr Ofni could still edit her original schedule in EPED to produce the final variable list. She could also add other text either after the hash symbols or below to help with her coding. For example, she might type: *male=1*, *female=2* on the rest of the line which starts Sex #.

The template is saved by pressing F2 and choosing the option 'Save file to …'. The program prompts for a filename. It offers the default sub-directory (which can be changed on the opening screen). Dr Ofni decides to save it to a floppy disk in drive A:. She therefore types *A:DIABETES.QES*. The final three letters are important to identify the file as a template. She could have chosen any name and saved it to any drive or sub-directory but she had to append the QES suffix. She now leaves EPED by pressing F10. This returns her to the opening menu.

She has now completed the first step. The template file is successfully saved and she is ready to proceed to entering her data. If she changes her mind about the layout, the names of variables, or any extra text she wants to add, she can recall the file and edit it further. Alternatively, as the template is stored as an ordinary ASCII file she could retrieve it into her wordprocessor and edit it (or even create it) there. The advantage of using a wordprocessor is the increased sophistication and flexibility it offers: however, if you use one remember to save the final template with its QES suffix as an ASCII file as Epi Info cannot read the embedded formatting commands of ordinary wordprocessors.

Entering data

The next step is data entry. On Epi Info's title screen, Dr Ofni brings the cursor down to the program ENTER and presses <RTN>. She is prompted for the name of a datafile. This could take any name she wishes but as the template file was called DIABETES this seems like a consistent name. She therefore types *A:DIABETES* to place the data file on the same floppy disk as the template file. The program automatically gives the new file the suffix REC to indicate it is a record file. Pressing the <ESC> key acknowledges that this file will be created. Now the program prompts for the template file—which in this case will be the one just written. Dr Ofni enters here the address and name of this file, namely A:*DIABETES*. The QES suffix is unnecessary at this point as the program automatically searches for the appropriate file.

Having chosen the A:DIABETES.QES file the program puts Dr Ofni into data entry mode. On the screen she sees the template that she designed earlier, together with boxes awaiting her data.

Dr Ofni has already created a coding frame for her data:

Number   Code the actual number.

Age   Enter the two digits of the patient's age; remember that patient's under the age of 10 should be given a leading 0 (e.g. 06).

Sex   Code the patient's gender using the numbers 1 and 2 to represent males and females.

RBG   Enter the random blood glucose of the patient to one decimal point. Notice again that if the glucose is less than 10 a leading 0 (e.g. 05.7 will be needed.

Feet   Whether the patient's feet were inspected at the consultation is entered for the next question by using 1 to represent yes and 2 to represent no.

Dr Ofni then proceeds to enter her data. You might like to enter data for an imaginary patient. As you will see, the cursor moves automatically from question to question as you complete the answer boxes. You will then see an option at the bottom of the screen to write this data to your disk. By pressing Y (for yes) the data is entered into your DIABETES.REC file ready for analysis. The screen then offers a new template for the next case to be entered. You should similarly imagine another patient and fill in the responses, saving this in the same manner. Repeat this process ten times to create a datafile containing ten cases. When you have finished press F10. This completes the second step.

Data analysis

Now, from Epi Info's title screen choose the ANALYSIS program and press <RTN>. The ANALYSIS screen is divided into an upper output section and a place for commands to be entered at the bottom. The list of available commands can be obtained by pressing F2. The first command to use is READ. Press F2, place the cursor over READ and press <RTN>. You now need to write the name of your record file. For example, if this is on your C drive in the DATA sub-directory, type C:\DATA\FILENAME.REC. If you have been following Dr Ofni's work you would type A:DIABETES.REC, then <RTN>.

The program now reads the data file. The name of the file and the number of cases read is indicated on the top line of the screen. The data are now ready for analysis. Start with an examination of the overall distribution of each variable:

this requires the frequencies command. Press F2 to see a list of available commands and choose *freq* followed by <RTN>. Type * to denote that you wish to see the frequencies of all the variables in the study; press <RTN> to see the results. You will see the frequencies of the case numbers set out in terms of their numbers and percentages together with a sum, mean, and standard deviation. By pressing any key you will see each of the other variables in turn. Of course by simply typing *freq* and then *age*, you could see the age data alone.

Now press F2 and move the cursor over TABLES (or type the word *tables* at the command prompt at the bottom of the screen), and press <RTN>. Press F3 to see a list of the five variables in your data set. Move the cursor over SEX, press <RTN>, press F3 again and choose FEETINSPEC and press <RTN>. You have now constructed a command to produce a table of the sex of the patient by whether or not their feet were inspected. Press <RTN> to run the command. You will see the table produced together with accompanying statistics including the well-known chi-squared (see next chapter).

The available commands will also produce graphics. Press F2 and choose HISTOGRAM <RTN>. Now type (or choose from the variables list) *age* and <RTN>. You will now see a histogram of the ages of the patients in your sample. Press <ESC> to return to the analysis screen. Note that if you now wanted to produce a pie chart of age you could recall the previous command by pressing the 'up' cursor anew and editing it. Previous commands are saved 'behind' the output screen and can be recalled by using the cursor.

There are a number of other analysis commands which you will find useful: pressing F1 will provide a list of all the commands and brief descriptions of each. Note the ROUTE command which allows you to direct the output of your analyses from the screen to either a named file (to edit later using a wordprocessor) or to a printer. (For example: ROUTE A:DIABRESU.LTS or ROUTE PRINTER.) There are also some commands to enable you to manipulate your variables. An example is given below to illustrate how you might use 'age' and 'feetinspec' to create a 2 × 2 table.

Given that the ages you have selected are likely to span a wide range, any table produced is likely to be large (especially if you were to have a large number of cases). One means of coping with this is to create a new variable, say, AGEGROUP, and to assign it values dependent on the different age you wish to see. Thus:

DEFINE AGEGROUP #
LET AGEGROUP = 0
IF AGE >= 40 THEN AGEGROUP = 2
IF AGE < 40 THEN AGEGROUP = 1
TABLES AGEGROUP FEETINSPEC

Fuller descriptions of these commands are available via the help (F1) command, but briefly:

• DEFINE AGEGROUP # creates a new variable with one digit, in the same way that the template defined variables

- LET AGEGROUP = 0 places the value 0 in each of the empty # cells
- IF AGE >= 40 THEN AGEGROUP = 2 and IF AGE < 40 THEN AGEGROUP = 1 effectively makes the new variable a subdivision of AGE. It would have been possible to recode the variable AGE itself by using the RECODE command (RECODE AGE 1– 39 = 1 else = 2) but this would have meant that if later you wanted to look at individual ages they were lost from this analysis as they were recoded into only two groups.

Another command that is particularly useful is SELECT. Typing *SELECT SEX = 1* will ensure that subsequent commands are only performed on the males in the sample. Additional criteria can be specified. Thus SELECT BLOODSUGAR > 10.0 will identify only men with high blood sugars for subsequent analyses or graphics. Note that the selection criteria are described at the top of the ANALYSIS screen. The SELECT command is turned off by typing SELECT <RTN>—without any conditions indicating that all cases should be selected.

Further guidance in using ANALYSIS can be obtained by running the two tutorials provided with Epi Info. Type *RUN TUTOR1* or *RUN TUTOR2* from the command line in the ANALYSIS screen to see them.

Under the TABLES, MEANS, and REGRESS commands in the ANALYSIS program there are a number of statistical tests available. These include chi-squared, T-test, Mann–Whitney *U*, analysis of variance, correlation, and regression. Details of what these mean are given in the next chapter.

Other programs

EPED, ENTER, and ANALYSIS are the three basic programs that you are likely to use in general practice. However, the other programs in the suite may also be of interest.

1. CHECK provides support for data entry by ensuring that only 'legal' values can be entered. Open the program by placing the cursor over CHECK and pressing <RTN>. At the prompt, provide the name of a REC file. Try A:DIABETES.REC if you carried out the exercise above.

You will then see your familiar template as in the ENTER program, but with different commands at the bottom of the screen. Move the cursor to the SEX field and enter a 1. Now press F1. You have now stipulated that the minimum value that can be typed in this field during data entry is 1. Now type a 2 in the same field then press F2: this sets the maximum value as 2. If you were now to leave the program (saving the file when invited to) and return to ENTER you would find that the values other than 1 or 2 would not be accepted in the SEX field. This can be very helpful when entering data yourself or when you have asked someone less familiar with the data and coding frame. Errors in terms of illegal values are trapped before they are entered and the puncher given another chance to correct the mistake.

CHECK has a number of other facilities to help with data entry, such as jumping to another field if a certain value is entered in a different field, though the minimum/maximum value constraints are probably the most useful.

2. STATCALC provides both an estimate of sample size and the option of entering aggregated data directly into a two by two or three by two table. Open STATCALC in the usual way. Choose the 2×2, $2 \times n$ table option. Assume that you have completed a survey of whether boys or girls are more likely to get antibiotics for URTIs. Your receptionist added up the figures and found that out of 43 boys 16 had antibiotics and out of 51 girls 25 had antibiotics: is this difference significant?

Let the top line of the table be for the boys and the first column for a prescribed antibiotic. This means you should enter 16 in the top left cell <RTN>. Then 27 (that is, 43−16) in the top left cell. The second row is completed in the same way with the numbers 25 and 26. Pressing F4 will now provide statistics for the table. In this instance the chi-squared test (see next chapter) was not significant, suggesting that the observed difference was just a chance finding.

3. CONVERT and IMPORT allow data to be read into Epi Info from other programs (as indicated in the right-hand menu panel) and exported to other programs.

4. MERGE allows two separate REC files to be joined together.

5. VALIDATE enables two REC files to be compared. If resources permit, data can be punched in twice into two separate files. These files can then be compared for errors. Clearly the chances of typographical errors slipping through this procedure are very small.

Epi Info includes a number of other facilities that are of particular value to epidemiologists. Many of these can be accessed from the EPED program, and from there pressing F3 to run Epiaid. The programs in this suite will even design a study for you as well as semi-automatically creating an appropriate questionnaire for investigating communicable disease outbreaks!

An official manual for Epi Info is available at a reasonable price. It covers the information given in the F1 help screens together with details of other facilities (such as automated report writing). It even invites you to photocopy it and distribute it to your colleagues: how can you live without it?

SUMMARY

This chapter has offered a brief overview of personal computers and the range of available software. For those with a PC and a copy of Epi Info there has been a description of how to get into this extremely useful program that will meet most, if not all, of your data analysis needs. You will be impressed both by the sophistication and user-friendliness of this free software. It is almost worth buying a PC just to run this program.

9 Using statistics

'Don't be a novelist—be a statistician, much more scope for the imagination.' Mel Calman.

The initial exploration of the data will produce ideas about interesting relationships, some very clear, others suggestive. The task now is to determine whether the relationships between variables are as significant in the statistical sense as they seem to be when they are 'eyeballed'. In other words, those excess prescriptions given to adolescents may turn out to have no more importance than a chance variation, whilst the apparent small difference between prescribing rates to male and female elderly may turn out to be an important and 'real' finding.

How then should you set about examining the relationships between variables in a critical way so that the apparent will be separated from the real? The answer is easy—ask a statistician!

But just in case you do not have your own personal member of this quixotic species sharing the kitchen cupboard with your friendly bank manager, this chapter will describe the role of statistics in research. The subject of statistics often frightens people: it can seem very complicated and mathematical. But the logic of it is a lot easier than the complex formulae and sums suggest (which machines do for you these days anyway). Skim read this chapter at first: the best time to learn about statistics is when you have some of your own data and a question to answer.

This chapter will provide an overview of where statistics fits in the research process by describing some of the basic tests used—and employing as little mathematical knowledge as possible. At the end of the chapter you will have some idea of:

- which test to use in your individual specific circumstances
- when to use certain tests in general.

Hopefully this will be a true 'Duffer's Guide to Statistics'.

THINKING STATISTICALLY

Generally speaking there are two main ways by which a knowledge of statistics can help organize, sort through, and manipulate data that have been collected. Firstly, some way is needed of *describing* the data. All the facts and figures that are collected in a project appear to say many things but it is very difficult to see the wood for the trees. *Descriptive statistics* give a variety of ways of presenting and summarizing the information collected so that it is intelligible to a third party.

However, research is about asking and trying to answer questions. Very often data have only been collected from a sample drawn from a larger population so as to infer from the small to the large. The second branch of statistics, *inductive* or *inferential* statistics, can be used to look at some of these areas. It is based on probability theory and allows estimates to be made from the data that have been collected of how likely it is that the findings relate to the population from which the sample was drawn, or how likely it is that any hypothesis has been disproved. It uses more sophisticated, not to say at times convoluted, mathematical reasoning but is a vital tool in research.

Let us first look at various ways of organizing and presenting data.

NORMAN'S PROJECT

Dr Norman Curve, late of Puddletown Health Centre, now ensconced among the rolling hills of single-handed rural practice, has decided to screen a sample of 35–40 year olds for risk factors commonly associated with coronary artery disease. He wants to know how common are these 'common' risk factors, and whether they are associated with any other characteristics of the patient. He is particularly interested in knowing whether it will be worth screening both male and female populations. He therefore takes a random sample of 50 men and 50 women patients and invites them for screening. He decides to measure the following variables:

Concept	Indicator
Socio-economic status	Social class of main wage earner in household
Amount of exercise	Self report: nil–professional athlete
Smoking	Self report: Yes/No
Blood pressure	Systolic blood pressure
Amount of stress	Self report: 1–4
Overweight	Body Mass Index

The results from his sample are shown in Table 9.1.

QUESTION 9.1

How should Dr Curve represent the data to illustrate comparisons between the men and women in the sample for:

- social class
- systolic blood pressure
- amount of exercise taken?

Table 9.1 *Data set*

	Men						Women				
Social class	Exercise (0–4)	Smoking	Systolic BP	Stress (1–4)	Weight BMI	Social class	Exercise (0–4)	Smoking	Systolic BP	Stress (1–4)	Weight BMI
3	1	N	120	2	23	2	3	Y	120	1	20
2	3	N	120	1	20	3	0	N	130	2	26
2	1	Y	120	1	23	3	2	N	125	3	19
3	4	N	110	1	25	9	1	Y	120	1	27
3	2	N	120	2	23	3	1	Y	130	2	19
3	3	N	120	2	31	3	2	N	120	3	31
3	0	N	140	4	25	3	0	N	130	2	20
3	0	N	130	1	23	2	1	N	115	2	19
2	3	N	140	3	24	2	0	N	130	2	18
2	0	N	120	1	25	3	1	N	125	2	24
1	0	Y	130	1	29	3	0	Y	120	2	22
3	0	Y	130	1	25	2	2	Y	110	3	20
4	3	Y	115	1	26	3	2	N	120	1	20
3	1	N	120	1	20	2	0	N	130	2	25
4	2	Y	110	2	26	3	1	Y	120	2	22
3	0	N	120	2	28	3	2	N	110	1	34
3	0	N	135	3	24	1	2	N	120	1	20
3	3	N	120	3	23	3	3	N	120	1	23
3	3	N	125	1	20	3	2	Y	120	1	25
2	3	Y	120	2	27	2	0	N	125	1	25
3	0	Y	110	1	25	9	1	Y	120	2	21
3	3	N	120	1	25	3	3	N	130	3	24
4	3	N	125	2	26	4	0	N	110	3	26
1	1	N	135	1	25						19
1	1	N	130	2	24						23

Table 9.1 (*cont.*):

	Men						Women				
Social class	Exercise (0–4)	Smoking	Systolic BP	Stress (1–4)	Weight BMI	Social class	Exercise (0–4)	Smoking	Systolic BP	Stress (1–4)	Weight BMI
2	0	N	130	2	25	3	2	Y	120	2	25
2	3	N	130	1	23	3	0	N	125	3	22
3	0	N	125	2	22	3	3	N	120	2	21
4	3	N	130	4	30	2	1	N	155	2	26
3	2	N	120	1	25	3	3	N	120	2	27
3	0	Y	160	2	24	1	1	Y	120	1	18
2	0	N	130	1	21	3	3	Y	125	2	23
3	0	Y	145	3	28	3	3	Y	140	2	21
2	0	Y	150	1	22	2	0	N	120	2	23
2	2	N	150	2	23	2	0	Y	140	2	21
3	3	Y	140	3	25	2	2	N	125	1	20
2	0	N	150	2	24	3	1	N	140	2	21
1	4	Y	120	2	25	4	0	Y	125	2	26
3	0	N	125	2	26	3	0	Y	120	2	24
3	2	N	130	1	25	2	2	N	140	2	21
3	0	Y	130	2	25	1	2	N	135	1	25
3	2	Y	110	1	29	3	0	Y	145	2	29
2	0	N	125	1	20	4	0	Y	140	2	28
3	1	Y	125	1	27	3	2	N	130	2	23
4	2	N	120	1	25	2	3	N	120	3	23
2	1	N	110	1	23	3	2	N	130	1	21
3	0	N	120	2	25	3	0	N	140	1	21
2	3	Y	120	1	24	3	3	Y	120	1	27
2	0	N	120	1	21	3	1	Y	130	1	22
3	2	Y	145	1	26	2	3	N	140	2	21

Table 9.2

	Social classes					
	I	II	III	IV	V	E.I.
Men	4	15	26	5	0	0
Women	3	13	29	3	0	2

Social class

Dr Curve needs to introduce some sense of order into the apparent chaos of his raw data. The first task therefore is to compile a *frequency distribution table*. He does this by compressing the data into summary categories. In the case of the social classification this would naturally fall into the five social classes (I–V), plus a group for the 'economically inactive', coded as '9'. This would produce Table 9.2.

To some extent, the way the information is categorized will depend on the *level of measurement* chosen for each variable (see Chapter 7). Are the data at the nominal, ordinal, or interval level of measurement? If it is interval it is also necessary to know whether the scale of measurement is discrete, i.e. clearly defined differences such as number of children in a family, or whether it is continuously variable as with height, weight, or blood pressure. The number of categories chosen to summarize the data will therefore depend on the conciseness of the measurement on the one hand, and the clarity of the proposed chart on the other.

Perhaps a clearer way of representing the data above would be by means of a *bar chart*. The height of each bar represents the number in each group. (This is not to be confused with a *histogram* where the *area* enclosed by each rectangle is proportional to the frequency being illustrated.) When showing a comparison between groups, use can be made of shading or colour to distinguish between them.

Systolic blood pressure

Again the first thing to do would be to construct a frequency distribution chart. From the raw data in Table 9.1, it appears that the measurement was done to the nearest 5 mm of mercury, so that initially this could be taken as the class interval, producing Table 9.3.

A bar chart could then be used to illustrate the differences between the two samples (Figure 9.1).

An alternative method of illustrating the data might be to produce a cumulative frequency curve, also known as an *ogive* (Figure 9.2).

In this, the number in each group is added, going up the range. In our example the number of men with a systolic blood pressure of 110 would still be 5, but for

Table 9.3

Systolic BPs

	110	115	120	125	130	135	140	145	150	155	160	165
Men	5	1	17	6	10	2	3	2	3	0	1	0
Women	0	3	1	20	7	9	1	7	1	0	1	0

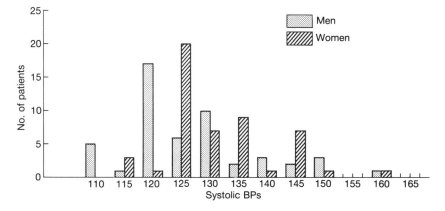

Fig. 9.1 Bar chart of systolic BPs.

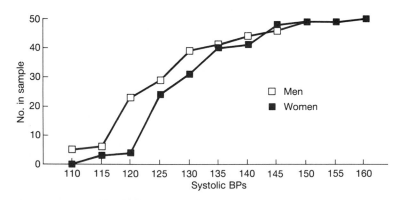

Fig. 9.2 Cumulative frequency curve of BPs.

Table 9.4

	Amount of exercise taken				
	0	1	2	3	4
Men	20	7	8	13	2
Women	15	11	14	10	0

Table 9.5 *Amount of exercise taken by the men*

Amount	0	1	2	3	4
Number	20	7	8	13	2
Degrees	$\dfrac{360 \times 20}{50}$	$\dfrac{360 \times 7}{50}$	$\dfrac{360 \times 8}{50}$	$\dfrac{360 \times 13}{50}$	$\dfrac{360 \times 2}{50}$
=	144	50	58	94	14

115 would be 1 plus the 5 already counted, and for 120 would be 17+1+5 and so on. Demonstrating the data in this way makes it easier to answer questions such as 'How many of the sample had systolic pressures below 130?', or 'At what systolic blood pressure were half the sample above and half below the figure?'.

Amount of exercise taken

As before, the first task to complete is to construct a frequency distribution table (Table 9.4).

Here there are only five categories, and possibly the clearest way of demonstrating the data is with a couple of *pie charts*—circles divided into sectors, one for each value of the variable. The area of each sector represents the proportion of the sample who have that particular value. These are particularly easy to construct using commonly available graphics packages for personal computers but they can also be constructed by hand.

In the present example, there are five possible values, 0–4, for the amount of exercise taken. Two circles are needed, one for the sample of men, and another for the women, and each would be divided into five sectors. The size of each sector is calculated using simple arithmetic. The whole sample comprises 50 cases, therefore the complete circle represents 50 cases. There are 360 degrees in a circle, and so in this example one case would be depicted by 360/50 degrees. Each sector size can thus be found by multiplying the number of cases holding that particular value by the proportion of the circle representing one case. This is illustrated in Table 9.5.

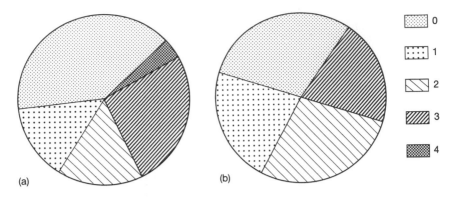

Fig. 9.3 Pie charts of exercise taken.

A pie chart could now be drawn, together with the corresponding one for the sample of women (Figure 9.3).

It is clear that there are various ways in which the data can be displayed to illustrate points or to highlight and suggest differences. The method chosen will depend on how the results have been classified, and especially on the number of categories into which the data have been placed.

EXERCISE 9.1

Construct tables and charts to present and contrast the results from the two samples for:

- smoking behaviour
- self assessment of stress factor
- ideal weight distribution.

Suggested answers can be found at the end of the chapter.

SUMMARIZING DATA

For many statistical tests one needs to develop a method of summarizing the values found for a variable—a kind of 'average' figure for all the data. There are two features about the data collected that are usually looked at in trying to summarize and describe the variable:

- a measure of central tendency
- a measure of the degree of dispersion of the data.

To give a simple example, if you were one of four partners in a practice and you were asked to describe the age structure of the partnership, but were only allowed to use one figure. You might add all the ages up and divide by four—this would give the *mean* for the data. This 'average age' might be 38. However, although very concise, this figure may hide the fact that the ages of the partners were 27, 27, 28, and 70. A measure of the *dispersion* of the data would give a third party a much clearer idea of the ages of the partners: 'My partners' ages vary from 27 to 70'.

'Might as well give all the ages in that case.' You're right. Giving all the results gives the most information, and is just as easy to do with only four cases to report. But when it comes to the 50 cases in Norman Curves's samples, or the many thousands that might comprise a sample in a large research project, one sees the need for summarizing the data. And not only are these summarizing statistics occasionally more convenient, but they are very important since they often form the basis of other statistical tests.

Measures of central tendency

The arithmetic mean

As we have seen, the mean or average is a commonly and easily derived figure. It is found by adding together all the values found for a given variable and dividing by the number of cases. So, in the data in Norman's screening project it is a straightforward task to calculate the mean systolic blood pressures for his male and female samples.

There were 50 observations for both samples. Adding the readings together for the men gives a total of 6345; when divided by the 50 readings, this gives a mean systolic blood pressure for the men in the sample of 126.9. Similarly the 50 systolic blood pressures in the women added together produces a total of 6305, and a mean systolic blood pressure of 126.1.

EXERCISE 9.2

Calculate the mean Body Mass Indices for both the male and female samples.

Suggested answers can be found at the end of the chapter.

The mean is a widely understood and easily calculated figure that takes into account all of the data within a group. However, as with the simple example of the partnership age structure, a few items of a very high or low value may result in the mean being a misleading figure in terms of representing the distribution of values within the group. For that reason, unless it seems fairly clear that the values are evenly and symmetrically distributed over a fairly narrow range, it may be better to choose one of the other measures of central tendency.

The median

The median is defined as the middle item in a distribution, that is the figure for which half the cases have a value less and half more. Obviously to determine the median all the cases in the sample have to be arranged in numerical order. If there happens to be an uneven number of values in a group then the median is the middle number. For example, if the four partners took on a fifth partner aged 56 the ages of the partners would now be:

27   27   28   56   70

In this series the median age would be 28 because there is an equal number of values (2) both below and above it in the series. If there are an equal number of cases in the group the median is conventionally taken as the mid value between the middle two. Thus, if the practice took on a sixth partner aged 35 the ages would now be:

27   27   28   35   56   70

The ages of the middle two cases in the series are 28 and 35. Therefore in this series the median value would be the mid point between these two values, 28+35/2 = 31.5.

QUESTION 9.2

In the screening project, what are the median values for the male and female samples for:

- amount of exercise undertaken
- amount of stress felt.

Since the sample size is 50 the median value will in all cases lie between the 25th and 26th values.

For the men, the amount of exercise taken by the 25th and 26th members of the sample when arranged in order is 1. Therefore the median figure for exercise in the male sample is (1+1)/2 = 1. In the female sample again both the 25th and 26th figures equal 1, and the median is also 1.

The amount of stress felt by the 25th and 26th members of the male sample when the figures are arranged in numerical order is 1, and again the median is 1. For the female sample both the 25th and 26th members of the series have a value of 2, and so in this case the median value for stress felt by the women in the sample is (2+2)/2 = 2.

EXERCISE 9.3

Calculate the median values for both the male and female samples for:

- systolic blood pressure
- Body Mass Index.

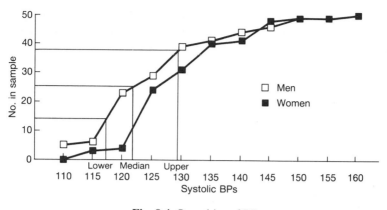

Fig. 9.4 Quantities of BP.

How do these figures compare with their mean values? Can you make any suggestions as to why they should differ?

> Suggested answers can be found at the end of the chapter.

There is another useful measure derived in similar fashion to the median. This is the *quartile*. As with the median, all the values for a variable in a series are ranked in order. The *upper quartile* represents that figure in the series which the top 25 per cent of the values in the series exceed, and the *lower quartile* has 25 per cent of the series with values less than it. Their relationship to the median can best be shown by using the cumulated frequency chart (described earlier): the relevant chart for the systolic blood pressure readings for men would show the quartiles and median as in Figure 9.4.

Note that the median is in effect the 50th percentile.

The median is often used when examining survival times, for example following diagnosis of cancer. The main reason for this is that the study need wait for only half the patients to die before producing a result, whereas it would need the survival times of all the patients if a mean was to be calculated. Similarly, in general practice, the median for, say, recovery time from an intervention is easier to obtain than the mean.

The mode

The mode again represents a type of 'average'. It is defined as the most frequently occurring value in a distribution, and the class with that value is called the *modal class*. A common use of it occurs when we talk about the 'average partnership having 3 partners in it' (even though the mean might actually be 3.124).

QUESTION 9.3

What is the modal class for the social class of Norman's two samples?

From the bar charts derived earlier it can be clearly seen that the modal class for both samples was social class III, which contained respectively 26 and 29 of the men and women in the samples.

Summarizing dispersion

Measures of central tendency describe the 'middle' of the data. Other figures are used to give some idea of the spread of results.

The range

This is the simplest way of describing a distribution. The range simply describes the spread from the lowest to the highest in the series. Therefore, using the four-partner practice described above, it is possible to say that 'the ages of the partners range from 27 to 70'. This certainly tells more than any of the measures of central tendency, and if used in conjunction with one of those measures would allow a fair guess at the underlying distribution.

The interquartile range

However, as in the above example, one or two extreme results might cause mistaken assumptions to be made. To avoid this, use is occasionally made of the interquartile range, which, as the name suggests, is the range between the low quartile and the high quartile met earlier. This, in effect, excludes both the lowest and highest 25 per cent of results.

QUESTION 9.4

What are the ranges and interquartile ranges for both samples for:

- systolic blood pressure
- Body Mass Index.

For the men the systolic blood pressures vary from 110 to 160, therefore the total range is 50. The interquartile range will lie between the 12th/13th readings and the 37th/38th. As the readings are 120 and 130, the interquartile range is 10. For the females the readings spread from 110 to 155, a total range of 45. The quartile figures are 120 and 130, and so, as with the men, the interquartile range is 10.

For the Body Mass Index the range for the men ran from 21 to 31, a range of 10, and for the women from 18 to 34, a range of 16. The quartiles for the men were 23 and 26, an interquartile range of 3. The corresponding figures for the women were 20.5 and 25, with an interquartile range of 4.5.

These various ranges give some idea of the dispersion of data around the central point, but can still mask the true *shape* of the distribution of the results. These shapes can be of many forms, but there are a few common ones.

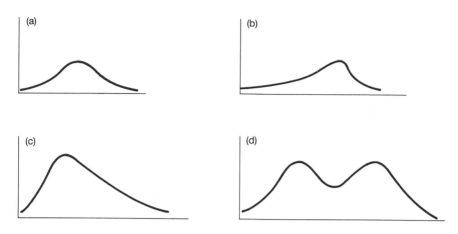

Fig. 9.5 Distribution curves.

In Figure 9.5 (a), the distribution of the frequency of occurrence of the results adopts a symmetrical shape, clustered around the midpoint, and the mode, median and mean all coincide. This bell shape, which can be found in many interval-based biological data such as height, weight, and blood pressure, is called the *normal* distribution.

Figure 9.5 (b) and (c) are examples where the results have clustered towards one or other extreme. These are called *skewed* distributions, negatively in the case of (b) where the clustering is to the right of the mean, and positively in the case of (c) where it is to the left.

The last distribution, (d), is an example of where there are two peaks in the distribution of the results—this is a *bimodal* distribution.

Obviously, none of the summarizing figures we have met so far will alone tell anything about the underlying shape of the distribution curve.

The standard deviation

Because the range and interquartile range are limited in their application, the *standard deviation* is often employed to describe dispersion, though it can only be used in symmetrical and unimodal distributions. It would be of limited value in either of the severely skewed distributions shown above, or with a bimodal distribution.

The standard deviation gives an idea of the spread of results around the arithmetic mean and hence gives an idea of the height of the curve. The greater the dispersion and spread of results, the greater the relative standard deviation, and the flatter the curve.

It also has other important properties. If the shape of the distribution curve is normal it is possible to show that 68 per cent of the results will fall within one standard deviation either side of the mean, and that 95 per cent of the results will

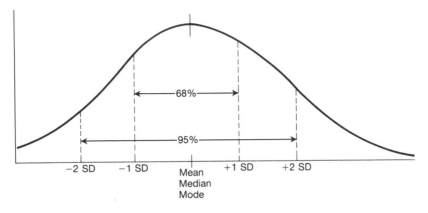

Fig. 9.6 The normal curve.

fall within about two standard deviations (actually 1.96) either side of the mean (Figure 9.6).

Therefore, if from the heights of the next 100 adult male patients the mean height was 1.62 metres, with a standard deviation of 4 centimetres, it is possible to say (since height is known to be a normally distributed variable) that 68 per cent of the adult males in the sample would have a height between 1.58 and 1.66 metres, and that 95 per cent would be between 1.54 and 1.70 metres.

The standard deviation is a measure of the dispersion of results around the mean and that is therefore how it is calculated.

1. The mean of all the results in the sample is calculated.
2. Each of the results is now taken in turn and the difference between it and the mean worked out.
3. Some of the results will be greater than the mean, and some less: some of the differences will be greater (+) than zero and some less (−). To remove the negative values, all these differences are squared.
4. These squared differences are added together.
5. This sum is divided by the number of results.
6. The square root of this figure is now taken to give the *standard deviation*.

Let us look at an example. You have joined your new partnership of five with ages 30, 35, 45, 53 and 62. The mean age of the partners is 45. This gives the figures shown in Table 9.6.

For each case in the series the difference between the value of the variable under consideration (age) and the mean for that variable in the series is calculated. If the deviations from the mean had been added together, the effect of the signs (+ and −) would have been to cancel each other out. The signs could have been ignored, the deviations added, and a *mean deviation* derived, in this case 50/5 = 10. It is more usual to square the deviation, in effect removing the sign.

Table 9.6

Age	Mean age	Deviation	Squared deviation
30	45	−15	225
35	45	−10	100
45	45	0	0
53	45	+8	64
62	45	+17	289

If the squared deviations are totalled they come to 678. This total, divided by the 5 cases, gives a mean squared deviation of 135.6. This figure is also known as the *variance*. The standard deviation is found by taking the square root of this figure, which in this example is 11.6.

The shorthand or formula which describes this process of calculating the standard deviation is:

$$S.D. = \sqrt{\frac{\Sigma x^2}{n}}$$

where S.D. represents the standard deviation, Σx^2 represents the sum of the squared deviations from the mean, and n is the number of items in the series.

A relatively inexpensive scientific calculator will do the actual calculation for you.

QUESTION 9.5

Calculate the standard deviation for the systolic blood pressures in the male sample.

Enter the values of the systolic blood pressures into a scientific calculator. The variance is 162.2 and standard deviation is $\sqrt{162.2}$, which equals 12.7.

If it were assumed that the results were normally distributed, then 68 per cent of the results would fall within one standard deviation of the mean, that is in the range 127 ± 12.7, say 114 to 140. In fact, 39 of our results do so, that is 78 per cent. Similarly, 95 per cent of the results should fall in the range 127 ± 25.4; 49, or 98 per cent of the results do so.

EXERCISE 9.4

Find the standard deviation for the Body Mass Indices for the two samples. Do you think they are normally distributed?

Suggested answers can be found at the end of the chapter.

MAKING DECISIONS—INFERENTIAL STATISTICS

As pointed out at the beginning of this chapter, descriptions represent only one limited use of statistics. Often it will be important to use the collected data to make some decision or statement about the population from which the sample or samples have been taken. In drawing a random sample from a population—say a one in ten sample of the over 65s from the age–sex register—it would be hoped that the sample will be typical of the whole population. But of course with some small samples chance biases can easily creep in. Yet the logic of the research is to be able to say something about the total population (i.e. all the ove-65s in the practice), and not just the one in ten sample. Statistics can come to the rescue here. They will allow an estimation of how closely findings from the sample are likely to reflect the population's actual characteristics without actually having to go to the often impossible length of measuring the latter.

On the other hand, it may be that the research involves comparing measurements from two samples and it is important to know whether any difference noted is real or whether it is just a chance variation to be expected when drawing different samples from the same population.

Chance and probability

Underlying many statistical decisions is the attempt to decide how likely it is that any one result can have been expected to occur by chance. Thus the chance that someone can guess your birthdate correctly would be one in 365, or 0.003. The probability that 'all men will die' is 100 per cent or 1.0. Usually probabilities are expressed in relation to this standard of unity. If an event occurs by chance one in ten times, it has a probability of 0.1, one in twenty 0.05, one in a hundred 0.01, one in a thousand 0.001 and so on.

In medical research the convention is that if the calculations show that a given result would have occurred by chance only one in twenty times, i.e. $p = 0.05$, then it is more than likely that this is a 'real' finding and not a fluke or chance result. For example, if a new hypotensive agent is found in a trial to reduce blood pressure by more than a placebo, it might be calculated that there was a one in twenty chance that such a result might be a random freak. However, the convention is to ignore this latter possibility if the chance is one in twenty or greater, and accept that it is the drug that is working rather than chance. In this case it is conventionally said that the result is 'statistically significant at the 0.05 level'. This attempt to quantify the likelihood that any given result or difference between results could have occurred by chance is all that most inferential statistical tests are about. At the end of the day they still make no absolute statements about the 'truth' or otherwise of findings. An unusual result that tests suggest would only have occurred by chance one in twenty times ($p = 0.05$) could still be that rare chance finding. Hopefully these issues will become clearer as the chapter proceeds.

The normal curve

The normal curve has been described above: what can you do with it?

The normal curve has one or two interesting characteristics, especially the fact that 68 per cent of figures in a normally distributed sample will lie within one standard deviation of the mean, and that 95 per cent will lie within two standard deviations of the mean. This can be used to make statements about an individual value in a sample, but more commonly it is used to relate the sample to the underlying population from which it was drawn.

The standard error of the mean

The concept of the standard error was briefly described in Chapter 2, when it was used to try and predict the size of sample needed in a particular project. You may remember that the mean of any one sample is unlikely to be exactly the same as the mean ('true mean') of the population from which it was taken. But interestingly, if a large number of samples were to be taken, it would be found that the results for the means of all these separate samples would tend to cluster around the true mean of the population in a *normally distributed* pattern. The standard deviation of this distribution of these sample means is called the *standard error of the mean*. Therefore, given that 95 per cent of all sample means from this one population will fall within two (or 1.96, to be precise) standard errors of the true mean, the result of the one sample that is usually available can allow a start in making assumptions about the underlying population with a known degree of mathematical certainty.

But hold on—how do you calculate the standard error of the mean for a population when you have only taken one sample? Surely you do not have to replicate your sampling exercise a dozen times?

Luckily it is possible to calculate the standard error from your one sample as long as you know:

- the mean of that variable in your sample
- the number of cases in your sample
- the standard deviation for that variable in your sample.

Armed with these results there is a formula (isn't there always?) that allows a calculation of the standard error:

$$\text{S.E.} = \frac{\text{S.D.}}{\sqrt{n}}$$

where S.D. is the standard deviation for that variable and n is the number of cases in the sample.

It is clear from this that the size of the standard error will depend on the size of the sample, as was pointed out in Chapter 2.

QUESTION 9.6

From a sample of 50 males between 35 and 40 years old drawn from the practice (Table 9.1), Dr Norman Curve established that the mean systolic blood pressure was 126.9. His practice list of 10 000 patients probably contains several hundred males in the 35–40 age group. What statement could he now make about the systolic blood pressure of all the males in the practice aged between 35–40?

He knows the following:

mean systolic blood pressure	126.9
standard deviation	11.4
number in sample	50

Therefore substituting into the equation above he can calculate the standard error of the mean:

$$\text{S.E.} = \frac{11.4.}{\sqrt{50}}$$

$$= 1.6$$

As a result of the characteristics of the normal curve he knows that the sample result of 126.9 will (nineteen times out of twenty) lie within two S.E.s of the true mean systolic blood pressure. In other words, there is a 95 per cent probability that the true mean systolic blood pressure of all 35–40 year old males in his practice will lie somewhere between $126.9 \pm (2 \times 1.6)$, that is between 123.7 and 130.1.

Since the standard error is inversely proportional to the sample size you may like to consider what he could have said about the true mean had the same results be obtained from larger samples of 100 and 200 patients.

With a sample of 100 the S.E. would have been 1.1, and so the true mean of that population of 35–40 year old males was likely (nineteen times out of twenty) to be in the range 124.7–129.1. A sample size of 200 producing the same results would have given a S.E. of 0.8 and so there would have been a 95 per cent chance that the true mean was between 125.3 and 128.5. Another way of saying this is that at the 95 per cent *confidence limits* the true mean lies between 125.3 and 128.5.

EXERCISE 9.5

Calculate the standard errors for the Body Mass Index for both the samples of males and females drawn from Norman's practice and displayed in Table 9.1.

What can you say about the Body Mass Index for males and females aged between 35 and 40 in your total practice population?

Answers can be found at the end of the chapter.

COMPARING SAMPLES

Often in research studies it is necessary to compare the results derived from two populations. For example, 'Does Skinnyfax cause weight loss over 6 months?' would involve comparing weight loss in a group of patients given Skinnyfax and a control group given a placebo. Or 'Is depression more common among women compared with men?' involves comparing depression rates in a male group with a female group. A useful way of recasting the question is to ask whether, from the results, the patients in the weight loss trial or the males and females in the study of depression are drawn from the 'same' population. In other words, if Skinnyfax has no effect it is as if patients receiving the drug were receiving the placebo— the two groups should be indistinguishable. Equally, if there are no differences in depression amongst males and females then, at least in respect of depression, it is as if they are all one population. Thus a finding that the samples are not from the same population suggests differences in terms of the factor (Skinnyfax and depression) under consideration.

It is usual to assume in the first instance that any differences that are found between the two samples have arisen by chance, and this is the reason that hypotheses are stated as *null hypotheses*. The research hypothesis may be that 'Skinnyfax causes a loss in weight', but for the statistical test the opposing null hypothesis is stated: 'Skinnyfax does not cause a loss in weight'. In other words, any differences in weight loss found in the treated and untreated samples are purely to be expected by chance. In short, any differences between the two groups can be explained by the expected distribution of the means of such samples (given their size and the usual spread of the variable being measured). However, if the differences found suggest that such results would be likely to occur by chance on less than one in twenty occasions then this suggests that the null hypothesis has not been supported. The hypothesis that Skinnyfax does not cause weight loss would be rejected (and by implication the conclusion drawn that it does cause weight loss).

Differences or associations?

The idea of the standard error is used to make statements about how likely it is that two samples have come from the same population. For example, 'Are men more likely to be overweight than women?' leads to a search to see whether there is evidence for a *difference* between the Body Mass Index for the male and female samples. Do they appear to come from the same population or is there evidence that they are two samples from different populations? Do children who clean their teeth regularly have fewer caries than those who do not wield the toothbrush? Has drug X caused a fall in serum potassium?

However, often research is trying to suggest more than that. It may try and show that the more there is of X the more of Y there is likely to be. This is the beginning of a more sophisticated statement of the relationship between two variables—not simply difference but degrees of association: *how much* is one variable associated with or changes with another, for example height and weight, number of cigarettes smoked and the incidence of lung cancer, socio-economic status and health. Not only might there be a difference in the amount of health between the 'rich' and the 'poor', but data suggest that the less of 'richness' you possess the less of 'health' you have. This task requires statistical tests that will measure that degree of association.

There is a battery of statistical tests and probably even more thin, thick, and very thick textbooks written about them. You may feel the need after this brief introduction to rush out and buy one, but in the meantime the following offers some basic guidance about deciding which test to use.

CHOOSING A STATISTICAL TEST

One limiting factor on the precise test that can be used will be the level of measurement of the variables being examined. Therefore, the first step is to ask: 'What level of measurement have I used for my variables?' Levels of measurement—nominal, ordinal, and interval—have already been described in Chapter 7. The lower the level of measurement the more restricted are the number of tests that can be used.

If the data have been measured on an interval scale then by looking at the frequency distribution curve for the data it is possible to ask a supplementary question: 'Are the data normally distributed?'. A useful way of then proceeding is to devise a simple table to summarize your data as in Table 9.9.

For example, for the question 'Are men more overweight than women?', the data could be summarized as in Table 9.7.

The question: 'Does systolic blood pressure increase with the degree of overweight?', produces Table 9.8.

If the measurements are not at interval level, or if there is doubt as to whether or not they are normally distributed then the tests that can be used are those suitable for *non-parametric* (i.e. not normally distributed) data.

Sometimes statistics textbooks offer aids to help in deciding which test to employ, usually in the form of a decision tree or table. Figure 9.7 is one such guide.

QUESTION 9.7

Dr Ashley Tension has decided to see whether people who smoke have higher blood pressures than non-smokers. His questionnaire asked the question, 'How many cigarettes do you smoke each day?' and the blood pressure of the sample was measured in mm Hg.

Which test could he use?

Table 9.7 *Data summary table (weights and sex)*

Variable	Value	Level of measurement
weight	BMI	interval
sex	M/F	nominal

Table 9.8 *Data summary table (weights and blood pressure)*

Variable	Value	Level of measurement
weight	BMI	interval
blood pressure	systolic reading	interval

Table 9.9 *Data summary table*

Variable	Value	Level of measurement

First construct a summary of the available data:

Variable	**Value**	**Level of measurement**
Smoking	Cigarettes/day	Interval—not normal
Blood pressure	mm Hg	Interval—normal

Following the decision tree, Dr Tension first asks 'Are both measurements interval?'. Obviously they are, so he can take the route to the left where he is next asked, 'Are both normal?'—that is, are both the variables being analysed normally distributed. Inspecting his data shows that since 60 per cent of his sample do not smoke the distribution curve of the number of cigarettes smoked in the sample is decidedly positively skewed. Therefore he answers no on the decision tree and this leads to the box which suggests that Spearman's rank correlation coefficient test would be the test to use at this level of measurement. As the name suggests, this is a test of correlation and attempts to show that a change in one variable is associated with a change in the second variable. Of course, there is nothing to stop him adjusting his level of measurement by reducing it to a lower level, for example by simply categorizing the response to the smoking

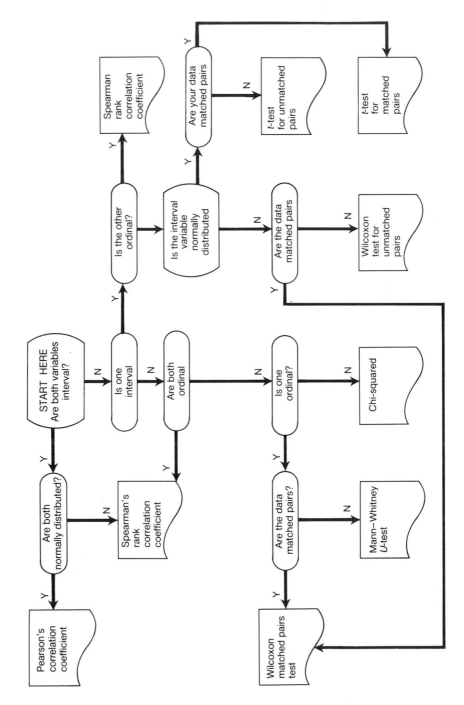

Fig. 9.7 Decision tree.

questionnaire into 'smokers' and 'non-smokers'. This would now mean that one of the variables was now at a nominal level, whilst the other was still interval and normally distributed. The decision tree this time would take the no path from Box 1, yes from Box 2, no from Box 12, yes from Box 14, no from Box 15, leading to the Student's *t*-test for unmatched pairs.

So why use Spearman's rather than the *t*-test? It is all a matter of the amount of information that one hopes to obtain from the data collected. Knowing that the amount of smoking is related to the degree of blood pressure, says more than just knowing that if you smoke you are more likely to have a raised blood pressure. By and large, the higher the level of measurement used, the more 'sensitive' is the statistical test that can be employed, and therefore the more likely that something interesting can be said about the nature of a relationship.

In the above example, Dr Tension could have gone one stage further down the level of measurement path and, for example, categorized the sample into those with blood pressure over 150 as 'high blood pressure' and those below 151 as 'low blood pressure'. His two variables would now be at the lowest level of measurement as both would be nominal. In a preliminary analysis of data it is often worthwhile doing this. By reducing data to dichotomous variables you can construct a 2 × 2 table (see Chapter 7) and apply a low-level test which, from the decision tree, you will see is the chi-squared test. In this way you should get a good feel for what the data set contains before applying more sophisticated statistical tests.

EXERCISE 9.6

In Norman's project, what tests could be employed to examine the following null hypotheses?

- The level of exercise undertaken by men is not associated with socio-economic status.
- Being overweight is not associated with perceived stress.
- Non-smokers do not exercise more than smokers.
- Smoking behaviour is unrelated to gender.

   Suggested answers can be found at the end of the chapter.

Some common tests of significance

Chi-squared

This is a very commonly used test of association. It can be used with any level of measurement but does require that the data categories are reduced to two or three for each variable, e.g. owner-occupier or tenant against income less than £20,000/year or more than £20,000/year. Typically data would be included in a 2 × 2 or 2 × 3 table. The basis of the test relies on calculating what the expected number of cases in each cell of the table would be if there was no relationship between the variables, and then comparing these with the observed result.

Table 9.10

	Stress < 2		Stress > 1	
	Expected	Observed	Expected	Observed
Men	21.5	26	29.5	24
Women	21.5	15	29.5	35

QUESTION 9.8

Is self-perception of stress higher in women?

This can be rephrased in the form of the null hypothesis: women do not perceive a higher level of stress than men.

From Norman's results we know that 24 (48 per cent) of the men admit to a stress score of more than 1, whilst 35 (70 per cent) of the women did so. Is this difference real or an artefact of the sampling? For the whole group of 100 men and women 59 (24+35) admitted to some degree of stress. Therefore, by chance it would be expected that 59/100 of the 50 men and 59/100 of the 50 women would admit to some stress. These *expected* results can be shown alongside the *observed* results in Table 9.10.

There does appear to be a difference. Fewer men and more women admit to some level of stress than one would expect. Is the result significant? To find out, use the chi-squared test.

The difference between the expected and the observed result is calculated for each of the compartments or cells of the table. This difference is then squared to remove the negative signs, divided by the expected result and these results are added together to give the chi-squared (χ^2) statistic:

$$\chi^2 = \frac{(21.5-26)^2}{21.5} + \frac{(29.5-24)^2}{29.5} + \frac{(21.5-15)^2}{21.5} + \frac{(29.5-35)^2}{29.5}$$
$$= 0.94 + 1.02 + 1.97 + 1.02$$
$$= 7.95$$

Now look up in a table of chi-squared values (found at the back of most if not all texts on statistics) to see whether this result is to be expected. To use the table you will also need to know the *degrees of freedom* available. This is a technical issue but easily calculated. The degrees of freedom in a table equals the sum of the number of columns in a table minus 1, times the number of rows in a table minus 1. In the example above, a 2×2 table, i.e. two columns by two rows, this means the degrees of freedom is $(2-1) \times (2-1)$, that is there is one degree of freedom for this table. In the table of chi-squared you will find that for 1 degree of freedom a chi-squared value of 7.95 would be found on fewer than one in ten

($p<0.10$) and more than one in twenty ($p<0.05$) occasions. It is therefore likely that the result was a 'fluke' and so the null hypothesis cannot safely be rejected. In summary, women in this study report more stress but not a *statistically significant amount* of more stress.

EXERCISE 9.7

Do people who exercise regularly (i.e. exercise score greater than 1) feel less stressed?

Suggested answers are to be found at the end of the chapter.

In summary, chi-squared can be used to show an *association* between variables whatever the level of measurement, as long as the number of categories for both variables is limited. It must also be remembered that chi-squared measures the significance of the association between variables, in other words it demonstrates whether an association exists, but makes no judgement about the underlying strength of that association.

Student's t-test

But what if the number of categories is not limited to a small number—how then do you draw conclusions about differences that exist between samples?

QUESTION 9.9

Are men in Norman's sample more likely to be overweight than the women?

The null hypothesis is that men are not more likely to be overweight than women.

Tabulating the variables as before:

Variable	Value	Level of measurement
Weight	Body Mass Index	Interval
Sex	Male/female	Nominal

The chosen index, the Body Mass Index, is an interval scale—the highest level of measurement. Looking at the frequency distribution charts earlier also leads one to suspect that the distribution of results does follow a normal-shaped curve. This allows use of more sensitive tests to explore whether the null hypothesis is supported or rejected.

The decision tree shows that the *t*-test for unmatched pairs could be employed. The *t*-test examines how much overlap there is between the population suggested by one sample and that suggested by the second sample. Do the figures suggest that the degree of overlap is sufficiently large to assume that the two samples are from the same population and that no true difference exists?

Mann–Whitney U-test

This is a non-parametric alternative to the *t*-test for unpaired data. It can therefore be used when one of the variables has been measured at an interval level but which is not normally distributed, or for data measured at an ordinal level. The other variable is measured at a nominal level. For example, one might be sex, i.e. 'men' and 'women' and the other 'number of cigarettes smoked per day'. The test is performed by looking at the relative *ranking* of the two samples as if they were a single population. The sum of the ranks in the smaller sample (if unequal-sized samples are being compared) is calculated and this can be compared with expected values for known sample sizes by looking at the relevant tables. If the figure calculated is greater or less than expected at the 0.05 level then one can say that it is likely that the samples represent different populations.

Matched pairs

In the decision tree you will have seen that one of the questions asked is whether pairs of data are matched or not. What is meant by this? Matching is built into the design of a project to eliminate as many possible 'hidden' differences between the samples as possible. In a simple 'before and after' design, the sample subjects are compared before and after an experimental variable has been introduced. In this sense the variable measured before is 'paired' with that measured afterwards, and so can be said to be matched. Another design may employ experimental and control groups that have been paired as closely as possible for as many variables as possible other than those involved in the experiment. Again the data from the two groups could be considered to be paired or matched. If the 50 men and 50 women in the study had been selected as 50 married couples then men and women could be compared by looking at these matched pairs. Using married couples would eliminate many socio-economic and other characteristics that might otherwise unknowingly have influenced the result.

There are two tests that can be used for data from matched pairs. One is the Wilcoxon matched pairs test that assumes a level of measurement slightly higher than ordinal, but can be used for non-parametric data, and the *t*-test for paired data, for normally distributed variables.

In the Wilcoxon test, the difference between the value of each of the pairs is calculated and then these differences are ranked, ignoring the sign of the difference. The sum of these ranks is calculated for the positive and negative differences. If the two samples are from the same population there is as likely to be a negative difference as a positive one, and so the sum of the negative ranks should about equal the sum of the positive ranks. The smaller of these two sums can be compared from tables for the known sample size (i.e. the number of pairs), and a probability for that figure found, thereby supporting the null hypothesis that both samples came from the same population.

Correlation

It is often possible to get the impression from the raw data that as one variable changes so does another. A correlation test will give an indication of the extent to which a change in one variable is matched by change in another. By how much will weight increase if height increases 10 per cent? How much more likely am I to contract heart disease if I smoke 60 as opposed to 10 cigarettes each day?

There are two tests commonly used to demonstrate and quantify the degree of correlation: Spearman's rank correlation coefficient for non-parametric interval data, or the product moment correlation coefficient (Pearson's) for instances when both variables being examined are measured on interval scales.

Spearman's rank correlation coefficient With this test the two variables are again ranked in order. If the two variables are not associated at all, then the rank of the second variable would be random and unrelated to the ranking of the first variable. On the other hand, if one of the variables was entirely dependent on the other then the ranks would be identical. Spearman's test gives a measure of how well the ranking of the two tests agree. This measure runs from −1, which suggests that as one goes up, the other goes down unit by unit, to +1 where a unit increase in one corresponds to a unit increase in the other. If there is absolutely no correlation at all between the two variables then Spearman's correlation coefficient will be zero. Again tables provide significance levels for any correlation coefficient: if, for example, there were 10 pairs a Spearman's correlation coefficient of 0.56 would only be significant at the 0.1 level—in other words there is a one in ten chance that the result could have occurred by chance. If, on the other hand, there were 30 pairs a correlation coefficient of 0.36 is significant at the 0.05 level.

Pearson's *r* can be calculated running from the same limits of −1 to +1.

Other tests This chapter has deliberately only looked at a small number of all the available tests that can be found in statistics textbooks and elsewhere. Some others commonly used are:

• *ANOVA* or analysis of variance, which allows more than two sets of variables to be compared.
• *Regression*, which tries to determine the extent to which each of many variables may contribute to the change in a single variable.
• *Factor analysis* which, from a stewpot bubbling with variables, tries to link together those that appear to be connected.

Remember that for most data sets there will be a number of different tests that can be applied, but the common ones described above will suffice for most situations.

SUMMARY

To many people, statistics represent a confused and confusing area. Exactly what test to use and how to carry out that test presents great problems. This latter aspect, how to do the test, is nowadays much easier with the fairly wide availability of sophisticated statistics packages for personal computers that will not only do the test for you, but allow you to manipulate your data between levels of measurement to allow a variety of tests on the same data (see Chapter 8).

Most often you are trying to indicate how likely it is that any differences between two variables you are comparing could have arisen by chance. In an ideal world you would have discussed your whole project with a medical statistician and geared the design of your project, including the type of question and level of data response, to answer a specific question for which a particular statistical test has been selected. This would include, in most cases, an opportunity to estimate the size of the sample required to confirm the degree of difference you are wanting to show at a pre-determined level of statistical significance. Statistics thus can assume a prominent role in the design of the project. Unfortunately this is not an ideal world. Medical statisticians still need to be sought out—departments of general practice would be a start, departments of public health in districts another possibility. Even if this has not been done and you arrive at the stage of data analysis there is still much you can do yourself: consider the research question, the level of measurement, and the type of tests available. And go forth and multiply, or divide, add ...

SUGGESTED TASKS

1. Carry out a one week audit of your appointments system, establishing for each patient, the gap between the time they would like to be seen and the time they do actually get a consultation. Prepare some tables and figures which summarize your results.

2. Carry out a one week audit of all your consultations, noting whether your patients are male or female. Ask a colleague (possibly one of the opposite sex) to do likewise and compare your results using chi-squared:

	male	female
Doctor X		
Doctor Y		

ANSWERS TO EXERCISES

EXERCISE 9.1

For smoking behaviour we would suggest a pie chart; for stress factor and ideal weight distribution we would suggest bar charts.

EXERCISE 9.2

The mean Body Mass Index for the men was 24.56, and for the women 23.02.

How did you calculate the sum of the Body Mass Indices? Did you add together all the individual scores, or did you take advantage of the work you had already done in categorizing the results? Using the latter the sum of all the Body Mass Indices would have been:

$(20{\times}4) + (21{\times}2) + (22{\times}2) + (23{\times}8) + (24{\times}6) + (25{\times}15) + (26{\times}5) + (27{\times}2) + (28{\times}2) + (29{\times}2) + (30) + (31)$

Always try to take the easiest route, and avoid duplicating work.

EXERCISE 9.3

• The median value for the men was 125 compared with a mean of 126.9. The median for the women was also 125 compared with a mean of 126.1.
• The median Body Masss Index for the men was 25, with mean 24.6, and for the women was 22.5, with mean 23.0.

For all these results there is fairly close agreement between the mean and median figures suggesting there is a degree of regular symmetry about the distribution of the results.

EXERCISE 9.4

The mean Body Mass Index for the men was 24.6 with a S.D. of 2.5.

For the women the S.D. was 3.3 around a mean of 23.0.

EXERCISE 9.5

The S.E. for the men was 0.4, and for the women the S.E. was 0.5.

The mean Body Mass Index for the men aged 35 to 40 in the practice is between 23.8 and 25.4 at the 95 per cent confidence level. For the women the mean Body Mass Index is between 22.0 and 24.0 at the 95 per cent confidence level.

EXERCISE 9.6

• Level of exercise is ordinal, as is social class. Following the decision tree leads one to Spearman's rank correlation coefficient.
• Weight (BMI) is interval and normally distributed. Stress is ordinal. Again the decision tree suggests that Spearman's is the test to employ.
• Smoking is nominal in this study, and exercise ordinal. The decision tree suggests that the Mann–Whitney U-test could be tried.
• Smoking and gender are both nominal. Chi-squared is the test suggested.

EXERCISE 9.7

The null hypothesis is:

People who exercise do not have a lower degree of perceived stress.

The frequency table looks like this:

	Stress < 2		Stress > 1	
	Expected	Observed	Expected	Observed
Exercise	9.3	23	27.7	24
No exercise	21.7	17	31.3	36

Chi-squared = 2.92. The degrees of freedom number 3. Tables of chi-squared show that this is not significant at the 0.05 level and so the null hypothesis is supported.

10 Writing up the research

The chapters so far have described in detail the various stages of the research process, beginning with defining a question for research and developing a research design, through to analysing the data collected in the study using a range of statistical techniques. This chapter now focuses on describing the various questions and issues that need to be tackled in writing up the research.

Dr Greatman has been investigating the relationship between the allocation of time in general practice and list size. He has carried out a survey of a random sample of 200 general practitioners working in the region. Fifty-five per cent of the general practitioners completed and sent back his mail questionnaire, giving an achieved sample of 110. These data have been coded and put on the computer. His analysis has shown that list size is modestly but positively correlated to both hours worked per week in surgery consultations and hours worked per week in all work-related activities. However, list size is inversely but once again only modestly associated with consultation rates, home visiting rates, and consultation length.

Dr Greatman thinks that his findings are important and interesting but how does he tell other people about them? He phones his golfing colleague, a partner at a local Health Centre, to give him the exciting news. His colleague mumbles 'Oh, how interesting' and rather deflatedly Dr Greatman puts down the phone. He could on the other hand give a talk to colleagues, but must he wait in hope for the invitation that never comes? Anyway this would only reach a small number of people. He decides that the only answer is to write up the results for publication in an academic journal; that way he will reach a wide audience and maybe achieve just a little bit of fame.

WHAT SORT OF DOCUMENT TO WRITE

There are two options:

- a report that contains a detailed account of the study and analysis of findings
- a paper or article for publication.

Reports are detailed descriptions of the study as a whole and tend to be required by grant-giving bodies to show what was finally produced with their money. However, its distribution is likely to be limited and it will probably be too long and detailed for people to read in any depth. It is therefore more usual to try for a publication, not just to be seen as clever and famous but because it obtains the widest possible readership. There are in addition other advantages of publication:

- publication in a reputable journal using scientific referees implies that the research is of good quality
- publication is crucial in the development of a research career and without publication it is increasingly difficult to make progress and gain further financial support.

Dr Greatman is aware that his paper might not be accepted for publication and he might end up with nothing to show for his painstaking efforts. However, he is also aware of the proliferation of new journals in the area and as a last resort feels—somewhat arrogantly—that he can always 'dump' his paper in one of the possibly less prestigious journals.

HOW TO STRUCTURE A SCIENTIFIC PAPER

The most common structure for a paper involves it being divided up into four sections:

- introduction
- methods
- results
- discussion (and conclusion).

Writing the introductory section

The introduction sets the scene for the study. It should include a brief review of the main literature in the area, citing and summarizing important earlier studies. This should be followed by a statement of the question which the research has tried to answer. The skill in writing the literature review is to get it to the point where the research question seems the next natural step. Alternatively, especially when there is little existing literature, a few sentences may be necessary to justify and explain the importance of the study.

Dr Greatman sits down with a gin and tonic that weekend after a visit to the library to write the first draft of his intended introductory section:

Draft: Smith[1] found little evidence of any variation with list size in the total number of hours spent each week by general practitioners in patient care. Jones and Marsh[2] found a similar pattern of evidence to Smith as did White[3]. Wilcalfe and Metkin[4] found a strong positive correlation between list size and the aggregate amount of time spent each week in surgery consultations and home visits. Swift[5] found little evidence of an association between list size and consultation rate and home visiting rate although the opposite pattern was found by Davis[6]. Wilcalfe and Metkin[4] found little evidence of an association between list size and consultation length.

This study further explores the relationship between list size and the allocation of time in general practice. This question is of importance because it has been argued[7] that lowering list sizes would lead to a better standard of care in general practice. This research therefore addresses one of the most important issues in general practice today and its findings should have far-reaching consequences in health policy in this area.

What are the major weaknesses in this introductory section?

1. It is better to move from the general to the specific rather than the specific to the general. Thus, the policy questions in the second paragraph about the impact of lowering list sizes on the standard of care might have been raised at the beginning of the paper putting the more specific research question in a broader context. It might also be necessary to spell out the assumed link between reduction in list size, release of time, and improvement in the standards of care.

2. The introduction should describe how the research links with the pattern of evidence and the development of the research that has been published previously on the topic. Thus, it is a matter of identifying the key research in the area to show how this previously published research supports or illustrates arguments in the paper. The major problem with the introduction as it stands is that the described research studies tend to duplicate one another. Also, the literature tends to lead the argument and the implications of the previous evidence for the current research study are not clearly drawn out.

3. The introduction should contain an explanation or explanations for carrying out the specific piece of work. No reasons are given in this introduction for why it was necessary to further examine the link between list size and the allocation of time. Why is this new research superior to that which has previously been carried out? What are its novel qualities? Does it deal with a question previously neglected in the research or does it attempt to overcome the methodological deficiencies inherent in previous studies?

4. The introduction should also contain a description of the specific objectives and propositions to be examined. No such description is found here: for instance, What is the relationship between list size and hours spent per week in patient contact and all work-related activities, consultation rate and home visiting rate, and consultation length.

5. The introduction should also contain a description of the general method of investigation, i.e. include a statement such as 'drawing on evidence collected from a survey carried out on a random sample of 200 GPs in a region, this study examined the association between …'.

6. The final sentence may reflect the researcher's pride in the work carried out, but scientific convention requires more modesty and an assumption that the reader will judge the importance of the study.

In summary, the introductory section should:

- begin with a broad issue or problem and move towards a more specific research question
- identify the key research in the area and use it to illustrate the paper's arguments
- identify the novel qualities of the proposed research and give explanations for carrying out this particular project

- describe the objectives of the study and the specific question(s) to be explored
- describe the general method of investigation
- not claim too much for the work.

Here is a rewritten version of the introduction which attempts to incorporate each of these points.

For several years the policy of the General Medical Services Committee has been that list sizes in general practice should fall to a target national average of 1700. This is usually justified on the grounds that smaller lists produce higher standards of care.[1] The key factor that is believed to mediate the relation between list sizes and standards of care is time; if general practitioners acquire smaller lists, the argument runs, they will have time to enhance the standard of care in their practices[2] through extending their consultation time.

In his review of published studies up to 1980 Butler found little evidence of any systematic variation with list size in the total number of hours spent each week by general practitioners in caring for patients.[3] The extra time available to doctors with smaller lists was much less likely to be spent on longer consultations than on higher rates of consultation in the surgery and home visiting. In their study of 199 general practitioners in inner and outer Manchester, Wilkin and Metcalfe[4] found a strong positive correlation between list size and the aggregate amount of time spent each week on consultations and home visits. This study did, however, support the earlier work[5] in showing that there is no more than a slight relation between list size and length of consultation and an inverse association between list size and the rate of consultation. Thus, it may be unrealistic to expect general practitioners to respond automatically to smaller lists by increasing their length of consultations.

There are, however, deficiencies in previous studies; they were often confined to self-selected practitioners, sometimes had low rates of response, and did not usually measure the allocation of time among all the components of the working week. In this study an attempt was made to surmount these deficiencies and a survey was carried out based on a random sample of GPs working in the region. The objective of the study was to investigate to what extent list size influences the amount of time a GP spends in work-related activities.

Writing the methods section

The methods section should present the method used with sufficient clarity and detail such that the reader would be able to replicate the study.

Now, satisfied with the introduction, the following Tuesday, after 'East Enders', Dr Greatman drafts out the next section:

Draft: The data collected in this study were derived from information gathered from 110 general practitioners working in the region. This information included data on personal list size, on booking interval, on consultation rate and home visiting rate and hours worked per week on a range of work-related activities. An analysis was carried out examining the relationships between personal list size and the indices of time.

What are the weaknesses of this methods section?

1. There is a complete absence of information about the research design and why a cross-sectional survey was used to test the specific proposition.

2. No information was given about the sampling frame, the sample size, or the method of sampling.

3. There is also absence of information about the method of data collection. A mail questionnaire was chosen with a reminder postcard 3 weeks later, followed by a reminder letter 3 weeks after the postcard. Any pilot studies also need to be mentioned.

4. There is absence of information about how the concepts were operationalized. How were the consultation rate and home visiting rate calculated?

5. There needs to be some observation about the reliability and validity of the measures used in the study.

6. There is an absence of information about the form of the analysis. What statistical tests were going to be used?

In summary, the methods section should contain:

- description of sampling frame, sampling method, sample size, and description of the design chosen
- description of method of data collection and how the instrument was piloted
- description of how the concepts were operationalized
- comment on the reliability and validity of any instrument
- description of techniques to be used in the analyses.

Here is a revised version of the methods section that attempts to incorporate these points.

The study was a postal survey of a non-statistical sample of unrestricted principals in the region. The addresses of the 200 doctors selected were obtained from the FHSA lists. The first mailing was sent in October 1992, and two follow-up mailings were used.

Seven characteristics were obtained for most of the non-responders as well as the responders: year and place of qualification, sex, whether they were members of the RCGP, personal list size, average list size in the practice, and geographical location. All the data were collected through a self-completed questionnaire; the questions had been piloted in a small study of trainers ($N = 20$). All the information collected was based on doctors' reports and was not validated from independent sources. The primary focus of the study was on the performance of individual GPs and so it was decided to collect information about the personal lists of the respondents in the survey.

Data from returned questionnaires were entered into a personal computer and analysed using EpiInfo. The statistical relationship between personal list size and the allocation of time was analysed using Pearson's correlation coefficient.

Writing the results section

The results section is where the findings are presented. The commonest failing here is to give too many results in too much detail. Remember that the reader does not have either the same intimate knowledge nor interest in every detail. Try and summarize. As an incentive, many journals restrict the number of tables permitted to about six.

Rain has stopped the golf club tournament so Dr Greatman takes the opportunity to write the draft of his results section:

Draft: Table 10.1 shows the distribution of the estimates of time spent per week in a range of practice based activities. The table shows marked variations in time spent on both surgery consultations and home visits which were the activities which made up the bulk of the working week for most doctors.

Table 10.2 shows the strength of the relationship between list size and the indices of time. The table shows that list size was negatively associated with booking interval, consultation rate, and home visiting rate but positively correlated with numbers of hours in surgery consultations and all practice based activities.

What are the major weaknesses in the results section?

1. If the study involves a survey then it is customary to lead with the response rate. In this study it was 55 per cent, which is quite low. It is then usual to compare responders and non-responders as far as possible to see to what extent the latter are a different group. Thus, for example, if they are found to contain more older GPs then any relationship between GP's age and other variables will have to be considered in the light of this bias. On the other hand, no significant differences between responders and non-responders gives some justification to the assumption that the latter would have replied like the former.
2. Table 10.1 contains a large amount of information and it would be much clearer if the table was broken down into practice-based activities and activities outside the practice, such as private practice.
3. Table 10.2 contains figures that are percentages rather than actual values and yet there is no mention of percentages in the table. Also, there is no information on sample size for each of the categories.
4. Table 10.2 presents a correlation matrix but there is no reference to the specific statistical test being used nor were there any details of levels of statistical significance.
5. Although the strength of the inter-relationships between the indices of time is of interest it is not directly relevant to this particular analysis. The aim here is to examine the strength of the relationship between list size and the indices of time. While the correlation is useful it might have been better to present these relationships in the form of graphs.
6. Some of the correlations were to five decimal places and others to four. It is better to have consistency throughout and four decimal places is probably sufficient.

In summary, the results section should contain:

• a statement on the response rate and any bias
• clear tables or graphs which do not contain too much information or irrelevant information
• a clear and concise commentary on the tables and graphs highlighting the major points

Table 10.1 *Estimates of time spent each week on all activities*

	None	1	-2	-3	-4	>4	≤5	10	15	20	25	30	>30	Mean number of hours
Surgery consultations	–	–	–	–	–	–	1	3	19	41	–	10	5	20
Home visits	–	–	–	–	–	–	20	45	22	10	3	1	1	10.5
Practice administration	–	–	–	–	–	–	85	13	2	1	1	–	–	3.2
Reading, research	–	–	–	–	–	–	87	11	2	1	1	1	–	2.9
Training courses	–	–	–	–	–	–	–	–	–	–	–	–	–	
Other	–	–	–	–	–	–	88	10	1	1	–	–	–	2.2
Private practice	83	10	3	1	1	2	–	–	1	–	–	–	–	0.4
Hospital appointment	70	2	4	4	6	13	–	–	–	–	–	–	–	
Insurance work	48	34	13	4	2	1	–	–	–	–	–	–	–	0.7
Clinic	77	6	10	3	2	2	–	–	–	–	–	–	–	0.6
Police and industrial work	84	6	4	1	2	3	–	–	–	–	–	–	–	0.5
Committee work	78	12	5	2	1	2	–	–	–	–	–	–	–	0.4
Teaching	91	5	2	1	1	1	–	–	–	–	–	–	–	0.2
Other	86	3	3	2	1	4	–	–	–	–	–	–	–	0.4

Table 10.2 *Interrelationships between list size and indices of time*

	List size	Booking interval	No. of hours in surgery consultations	No. of hours in all activities	Consultation rate	Home visting rate
List size	–					
Booking interval	–0.1941	–				
No. of hours in surgery consultation	0.2570	0.13638	–			
No. of hours in all activities	0.2034	0.06323	0.58919	–		
Consultation rate	–0.33842	–0.09077	0.12527	0.12046	–	
Consultation rate	–0.2004	–0.07448	0.01742	0.19420	0.19920	–

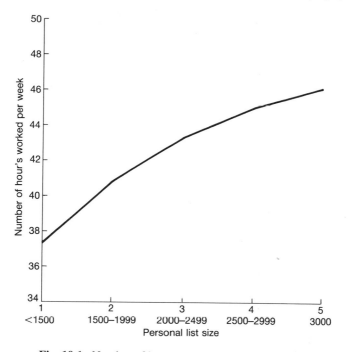

Fig. 10.1 Number of hours worked by personal list size.

- information about sample sizes, statistical tests used, and levels of statistical significance
- graphs and figures to illustrate the strength and nature of relationships between variables.

Examples of how the data could be presented are shown in the following tables and graphs. Tables 10.3 and 10.4 illustrate how to present the data about doctors' estimates of time spent on practice based activities (Table 10.3) and non-practice based activities (Table 10.4). The tables include both values and percentages and sample sizes for each activity.

Figure 10.1 illustrates how data can be presented in the form of a graph. It shows the relationship between personal list size and number of hours worked per week and gives a much clearer picture than just presenting correlations or tables.

Writing the discussion

The discussion section is where inferences from the findings are drawn and where conclusions are presented. There is often a tendency to put results in the discussion and vice versa. Try and keep them separate.

Table 10.3 *Respondents' estimates of the time spent each week on GMS activities*

| | Distribution of respondents' estimates | | | | | | | | |
	5 hours or less (%)	5.1 to 10.0 hours (%)	10.1 to 15.0 hours (%)	15.1 to 20.0 hours (%)	20.1 to 30.0 hours (%)	25.1 to 30.0 hours (%)	more than 30 hours (%)	n (=100%)	Mean
Hours per week spent on:									
Surgery consultations	1	3	19	41	22	10	5	1390	20.0
Home visits (including travelling)	20	45	22	10	3	1	–	1378	10.5
Practice administration	85	13	2	–	–	–	–	1410	3.2
Reading, research, training courses	87	11	2	1	–	–	–	1409	2.9
Other	88	10	1	1	–	–	–	1411	2.2
All GMS activities									38.8

Table 10.4 *Respondents' estimates of the time spent each week on non-GMS activities*

			Distribution of respondents' estimates				
	None	1 hour or less (%)	1.1 to 2.0 hours (%)	2.1 to 3.0 hours (%)	3.1 to 4.0 hours (%)	more than 4 hours (%)	n (=100%)	Mean
Hours per week spent on:								
Private practice	83	10	3	1	–	2	1413	0.4
Hospital appointments	70	2	4	4	6	13	1399	1.4
Insurance work	48	34	13	4	2	–	1377	0.7
Clinics	77	6	10	3	2	2	1406	0.6
Police industrial work	84	6	4	1	2	3	1347	0.5
Committee work	78	12	5	2	1	2	1391	0.4
Teaching	91	5	2	1	1	1	1385	0.2
Other	86	3	3	2	1	4	1394	0.5
All non-GMS activities								4.7

At last a break in a busy morning for Dr Greatman; the Placebo Pharmaceutical's representative has phoned to say his car has broken down: time to set out the discussion:

Draft: The results from this study clearly show that list size is strongly related to the time general practitioners spend at work. The results show that as list size decreased the doctors spent less time at work overall but increased their rate of consultation and rate of home visiting and increased the length of their consultation. These findings provide strong support for those who wish to see further reductions in list size. There is clear evidence from this study that a fall in list size will lead to doctors reinvesting the extra time released into improving existing care and developing new forms of care. Thus, future policy might concentrate on moving towards the General Medical Services Committee's target of national average list size of 1700 as this evidence suggests the pay-off would be a large one.

What are the major weaknesses in this discussion section?

1. The discussion and conclusions drawn from the study do not reflect the pattern of results that were actually found. The strength of the relationship between list size and any of the indices was never more than modest and in the case of home visiting rates was quite weak. Thus, the implication that list size was strongly associated with at least some of the indices of time is not entirely accurate.
2. The research design used was a cross-sectional one and the study investigated the relationship between variables. It is not possible using this kind of design to tell in which direction the causal relationship goes. Does list size determine hours spent in patient care or vice versa? To examine this question would need a longitudinal design as it would be necessary to find support for the conclusion that a reduction in list size would lead to a fall in hours worked and increase in consultation rate, home visiting rate, and consultation length. Perhaps a study using a longitudinal design should be a recommendation for further research. This type of recommendation usually comes in the final paragraph of the discussion.

In summary, the discussion section should:

- comment on the methods used, picking up their weaknesses (before the reader does!)
- contain a broad discussion of the findings that should include explanations for ambiguous or apparently contradictory findings
- contain the various possible interpretations of the relationship between variables
- show how far the findings are similar to or different from those found in other research projects
- discuss the implications of the key findings
- conclude with a statement of what the study has shown and, if appropriate, suggested directions for future research in this area.

Here is an example of how a revised version of the discussion might look which attempts to incorporate each of these points.

Despite the low response rate, comparison of non-responders and responders did suggest that the sample was typical of GPs in Britain. The times spent by GPs on various activities were estimates and therefore open to bias; however, the range of responses accorded with the findings of other studies, thus lending weight to their validity.

It has been argued that for GPs to be able to provide new forms of care or improve existing care they need additional resources, including time. Extra time can be created through further reductions in list size. Evidence from this study provided only partial support for this argument. The evidence suggested that personal list size was particularly important for explaining variations in hours spent in surgery consultation and surgery consultation rates. This finding corroborates evidence from other studies[3] although Wilkin and Metcalfe[4] found that the pattern was not consistent over the full range of list sizes.

The weakest relationship between the indices of time and list size was with consultation length. While there was a statistically significant trend it was not a strong one and this is consistent with other studies which have also shown the lack of any systematic association between list sizes, and average face-to-face contacts[6].

In conclusion, the evidence from this study suggests that while list size may be a key enabling factor in creating the conditions which give the general practitioners more time to spend, possibly in patient care or other work-related activities, it still does not fully account for variations in the allocation of time amongst these activities. The implications of these findings for policy suggest that the relationship between list sizes and doctors' behaviour is more complicated than is generally implied in the arguments about the beneficial effects of reducing the national average list size. Certainly, the evidence suggests that other changes are also required for doctors to change their behaviour and reinvest the time released from lower surgery hours into spending longer consultations with their patients.

COMPLETING THE MANUSCRIPT

The manuscript is almost complete but needs some additional information.

The abstract

The beginning of the paper needs to have a *title page* followed by an *abstract* or *summary*. The title page should contain the title of the paper, the names and qualifications of the authors, and the addresses of the authors, particularly for correspondence.

The abstract or summary is an important section that in some ways is the most difficult to write. It is important because it is sometimes the only section that is read by those browsing through the journal. The aim is to write a clear precis of why the work was done? How was it done? What were the findings? And what do the findings mean? Many journals now ask for structured abstracts in which the summary is provided over a number of sub-headings. The exact style can be established from the journal in question.

The presentation of the typescript

The text itself should be double-spaced with wide margins on right and left. It is customary to turn the right-hand margin justification on the wordprocessor into the 'off' position. This is because with the right-hand margin justified, breaks often appear in words as they are shuffled around to fill the available space and the printers who set the final text do not know whether these breaks are intended to be a part of the manuscript or not.

Acknowledgements

The end of the text may require an *acknowledgements* paragraph listing people who have made a significant contribution to the study, such as interviewers, secretaries, clerical assistants, advisers, and consultants. They should be acknowledged along with others who have made detailed and constructive comments on the paper. Financial sponsors should also be acknowledged.

References

The text finishes with a list of *references*. This can be one of the most irritating and annoying aspects of preparing a paper for publication. One of the problems is ensuring that you have the full details for all the literature that you wish to cite. If you do not adopt the practice of writing the references out in full when you have identified them then there is always the problem of remembering where you saw the paper, and so on. One way around this is to have a set of index cards on which references can be stored or use computer-based reference management software.

A further problem is *layout of references*. Different journals have different methods, although there is increasing standardization. Two different approaches tend to be adopted for the citing of references in the text. First, there is the Harvard system in which authors' surnames and date of publication are placed in the text in brackets. Secondly, there is the Vancouver system which uses numbers (either superscript or in brackets), and there are two variations of this system. The numbers may run sequentially through the text or be keyed to the list of references which is arranged in alphabetical order. The listing of references can, for both the Harvard and Vancouver systems, be in alphabetical order but, as with the *British Medical Journal*, might be listed in number order. The layout and arrangement of the references in the list at the end of the paper may also vary, and it is best to consult the journal before writing the references down. It is important that the layout of the references complies with the journal's style as, if it does not, it can unnecessarily irritate editors and delay publication. Some journals include the guidelines for the format of papers in every edition and others only include them in one or two editions throughout the year.

Tables and figures

The paper includes tables and figures. Each one should be presented on a separate page at the end of the paper, although their position in the text should be shown, for example by a blank space in which is written: 'Table ABC about here'. (This is to help the printer lay out the page in an attractive way.)

Revising the draft

Writers are seldom able to produce the final polished version of their paper at the first attempt. It is always better, even before sending it to co-authors or colleagues, to wait a week or so and then go back to revise and rewrite those parts that are unclear. At this stage it will be possible to check the structure and accuracy of the paper. When completed, it is useful to circulate the paper for comments from friendly colleagues and obtain agreement from persons quoted, collaborators, and sponsors. When the comments have all arrived it is time to re-draft, incorporating constructive criticisms. Once this is done the paper can be re-typed and shown to co-authors. When everybody agrees it is suitable it can be sent for publication.

GETTING IT PUBLISHED

On receipt of a manuscript the editor of the chosen journal will send an acknowledgement and send the paper off to scientific referees, experts in the field who are invited to read and comment on the suitability of papers for publication in that particular journal. This task is an unpaid one and sometimes experts in the field feel they have neither the time nor inclination to referee all papers sent to them: editors therefore sometimes have to try one or two experts before they find someone who will agree to take on the task. The number of referees used varies from journal to journal although it is seldom more than two. The referees chosen are usually those who have expertise in the particular topic or in the methods and techniques used, and editors usually try to select referees so that they can receive a balanced interpretation of the paper. Thus, if it covers medical and social aspects the editor may use a medical practitioner and a sociologist as referees or if it is medical and statistical a doctor and statistician will be used.

Depending on the journal, referees might or might not be told the author's name(s). Authors are never told the referees' names, though sometimes they can be guessed. In addition to giving comments about originality, technical quality, clarity of presentation and applicability to the area of the journal's interests, editors invite referees to rate the manuscript in terms of whether it should be published. These ratings tend to fall into four categories:

- accept without change
- accept with minor changes

- accept only with major revision
- reject.

The editor, on receipt of all the referees' comments, will make a decision and send his or her verdict to the author usually with either the full comments or extracts of referees' comments.

THE POLITICS OF PUBLICATION

It must be remembered that the process of gaining publication has a 'political' side to it that will soon be apparent when you get on board the publication ego trip. Here are a few pointers for when you are thinking about submitting your paper for publication.

The idea that journals are open and impartial in their judgements about what constitutes good research is not entirely true. If you are keen to get your paper published in a specific journal it might be sensible to have a look through the journal to see the type of article that it favours. Some journals do not like qualitative research and others which are a professional group's house journal tend to favour papers that do not criticize the policy of the professional association.

In some cases the author faces a dilemma. Do you submit your paper to the more conventional journal and water down the arguments for fear of rejection? Alternatively, do you leave the paper as you want it and submit to a journal with more radical views? The problem with the latter approach is that you are preaching to the converted. However, the process of gaining publication is usually a matter of negotiation between the authors, the editor, and the referees. In the end, it is important to be flexible and for authors to accept at least some criticisms and agree to some modifications.

If you are writing in an area where only one or two well-known authors have worked before it might be possible to predict who the reviewers will be. It might be possible to prepare in advance for the criticisms and try to incorporate defences in the paper. Some authors try to overcome possible adverse reviews by sending their papers around to other researchers before submission for publication. The aim is to take account of adverse criticisms before they are officially recorded. The obvious drawback is that having seen the paper in advance the reviewer may not feel it would be fair to review it and would advise the editor accordingly if asked to comment on it.

Publication has many idiosyncratic aspects to it although good-quality work, as might be expected, has the greatest chance of publication. However, the rule of thumb is to think carefully about the most appropriate form of publication for your work. Journals take several weeks if not months to make a decision about publication so choosing an inappropriate journal can waste a considerable amount of time and effort. It must also be remembered that the time lag between acceptance and appearing in print is seldom less than several months.

It is unusual for papers to be accepted at first submission. Referees and/or editors usually want some changes, even if only to grammar. There is, of course, initial disappointment that the paper was not accepted as it stood. But as if to rub salt into the wound the referees' comments often seem trivial or irrelevant. No doubt they sometimes are, but they always seem particularly carping the day you receive them. Read them a couple of days later and often you begin to wonder again if perhaps referees are human after all. Remember that refereeing papers, while it confers some power, is an unpaid, unacknowledged (because it is done anonymously) and time-consuming job, and that if someone has critically analysed your paper and written a page or two of comments they deserve some appreciation.

You will be advised of any changes required in a letter from the editor. This is usually accompanied by extracts of referees' comments to aid you in revision. If the editor's/referees' advice for change is very specific then, if you want publication, you swallow hard (it might be a favourite graph or sentence that has to go) and do it. Often however the advice is more vague: 'shorten the paper', 'sharpen up the discussion', or something like that. In these circumstances you try your best to achieve these goals and resubmit the paper. Depending on the extent of changes required the editor might or might not send the paper out again to the original referees to check whether you have made the specified changes. You might be able to influence this process if you include in your re-submitted paper a letter setting out point by point what you have changed in the original paper: a busy editor might accept your paper on the basis of this clear overview of what you have done without paying too much heed to the actual details.

What happens if your paper is rejected? Read the reasons given for rejection and in the light of these comments consider whether you should try another journal. There are a number of journals that accept material on research into general practice. Try each of the journals in turn (you will at least build up an interesting—and often diverse—collection of referees' comments). Then think about the GP 'comics': they need a regular flow of material, and while they do not count as a 'proper' academic publication (the mark of the latter is the expert refereeing process) they will pay you for your writing. The final alternative is to write your study up as a report and circulate it to colleagues.

EXERCISE 10.1

Identify the most appropriate journal(s) for publication of papers on the following topics:

1. a survey of patient satisfaction with the health service
2. an audit of preventive practices in three general practices
3. the prevalence of hypertension in a rural population
4. an evaluation of a health promotion facilitator in general practice
5. assessing methods of treating diabetes.

AUTHORSHIP

One of the most tricky aspects of publication is deciding on authorship. Obviously, this is not a problem if you do not have collaborators and you are the sole author. However, if others are involved, how do you decide who should or should not be co-authors and who should be the senior author (first author) who has the honour of always being cited (as in Einstein *et al.*). There are many 'grey' areas to this issue but the convention for allocation of the authorship status seems to be based on the nature of the contribution made by each participant. Those carrying out routine tasks such as coding might be acknowledged at the end of the paper. However, those who have contributed significantly in the form of ideas and creative thinking should be included as co-authors. The ordering of the authorship will depend upon the relative contribution made by each author. The person who makes the major contribution should be the first author (and that person, to earn the reward, usually writes the first draft, and co-authors then provide constructive comments and criticism). If the contributions are of equal proportion then the authorship is usually in alphabetical order.

SUMMARY

This chapter has concentrated on the writing up of the research. It has focused on issues and problems in writing a paper for publication and described the process of getting a paper published.

SUGGESTED TASKS

Go and read some journals. This time do not just read the abstract but note how authors have crafted their paper. Try to think critically: if you were asked to be the referee for a particular published paper what would you have written as advice to the author? (You are able to do this because papers, in a sense, are never finished, and even if published they could always have been further improved.)

ANSWER TO EXERCISE

EXERCISE 10.1

Suggested journals—there are no doubt more:

1. *Health and Social Services Journal*; *Journal of Public Health Medicine*
2. *British Journal of General Practice*; *Family Practice*
3. *BJGP*; *Epidemiology and Community Health*; *Journal of Public Health Medicine*
4. *BJGP*; *Health Education Journal*; *Family Practice*
5. *British Medical Journal*; *Lancet*.

11 Planning research

If you have not already started, now is the time to think about doing your own research. The previous chapters have covered a number of different skills you may require, though in the first instance you might like to start with something fairly straightforward such as a review of your workload. Then, when you see that research is not something restricted to ivory towers, you can be more ambitious.

THE RESEARCH PROTOCOL

For any research, even the most elementary, it is wise to prepare a statement about what you intend to do and how. This is more formally known as a *research protocol*. For a simple study it need be no longer than a page; it would start with a single sentence statement of the aim of the study and be followed by a paragraph or two on the precise method that will be used to achieve the aim. For a relatively simple study, such as establishing your prescribing rate over one week, it may seem that even this effort is unnecessary; however, it is a good discipline to get into and you will find that even with an uncomplicated study there will be times when a 'plan' is invaluable. In addition, putting things on to paper before starting can be very useful in identifying problems with the research. It is all too easy to sit in an armchair and imagine that the planned research is straightforward. Putting it on paper enables you to see if you have an answerable question and a viable method. Written plans enable you to show them to other people to get their comments and advice. This latter procedure is very important in working up any research proposal. A fresh eye, a different view, so often identifies silly errors or impractical plans, for even the most experienced researcher. Show your protocol to a partner, a spouse, or a receptionist, and ask them if it seems coherent and reasonable.

EXERCISE 11.1

Write a protocol to establish your referral rate over a one month period.

A suggested answer is given at the end of the chapter.

For research that is other than fairly basic you will need a more elaborate protocol. This will have various sections:

- title page
- introduction
- aims
- methods

- analysis
- funding requirements
- timetable
- references.

The first four sections are very similar to the initial sections of the research write-up described in the previous chapter.

First there will be a *title page* with the title of the study, the names of the researchers, and an address for correspondence.

Next there is the *introduction* that sets the scene and summarizes relevant literature. (*References* to the literature would be placed at the very end of the protocol.) Then follows a brief but important statement of the *aims* of the study, together with any specific research question(s) that it is intended to answer.

This is followed by details of the *method* it is proposed to use, specifically details of the overall design and sample. There is no need at this stage to include particular measurement schedules such as questionnaires: it is only necessary to say what form of data collection will be carried out. Details of the method are followed by a very brief overview of what you intend to do in the *analysis*. Of course, very often you will not know exactly what you are going to do until you have designed your schedules and collected and coded the data, so all you can be expected to provide is an outline of which variables you are going to relate to which.

Have you completed these sections adequately? The crucial thing to look for is the coherence of the aim, method, and analysis. The method, together with the analysis, should enable you to answer the questions advanced in the aims section. It is all too easy to add in an extra lump of analysis 'because you happen to be collecting those data': but if the analysis (or method) will help you answer questions that are not posed in the aims section that does not mean you have a 'bonus' but that either the aims, methods, and/or analysis sections need re-writing. The commonest mistakes in the early days of trying to write a protocol are that the method section will answer a different question to the one set out in the aims section, and the analysis will answer yet another. Read each of these sections carefully and ask whether they present a consistent picture.

Remember that the work you put in on these sections—perhaps several drafts as the ideas are pushed into shape—will be very useful when you later come to write up the research.

If your research plans are quite elaborate you may need to prepare costings so as to get an overview of your *funding requirements*.

Costings divide into several sections:

1. *Labour.* You will presumably work on the study yourself. Will this be 'spare' time or will it involve you in giving up clinical work and incurring locum costs? Will you need help with:

- clerical work
- secretarial work

- interviewing
- transcribing
- coding
- computing

2. *Equipment*

- stationery
- stamps
- photocopying
- telephone
- tape recorder
- printing
- computer

3. *Miscellaneous*

- travel
- conferences.

All of these costs should be carefully itemized even if you hope your study can be funded out of petty cash. Grant-giving bodies will expect the costs to be realistic.

The next page should be a rough breakdown of the timetable for the research. This is always difficult to estimate with any certainty, but the dates you do choose can act as a useful guide when you are in the middle of a project. Very roughly, research time can be divided into thirds: one third for planning and getting ready (up to and including Chapter 4), one third for the actual data collection (Chapter 5) and the rest for data analysis and writing up (Chapters 6 to 10). The actual details of a timetable are usually in months: for example, pilot study—March; data collection—April–July; analysis—August–October; and so on.

The final section contains the *references* from the introductory literature review.

RESEARCH FUNDING

There are various sources of funding for research available. Which one you approach will depend on the nature of your proposed study and your funding requirements. If it is a small scale study, with local relevance, and you need help with postage, stationery, and things like that, then you might consider approaching local bodies with immediate concerns for health service delivery. Local Medical Committees, Family Health Service Authorities, and Health Authorities may be willing to offer you small amounts to enable you to complete a piece of research which would have implications for local health care delivery.

If your research requires additional staffing—for example a research assistant or clerical officer—then this requires considerably more money. For this you are more likely to apply to a specific grant-giving body. The particular ones you might bear in mind are as follows.

1. The Royal College of General Practitioners Research Committee, which gives out several thousand pounds every year for research in general practice.
2. All NHS Regions now have Directors of Research and Development with the intention that these should oversee allocation of up to 1½ per cent of the total NHS budget to researching health care provision. Within this scheme, Regions may also have specific schemes for primary care research: it is worth enquiring.
3. The Medical Research Council has a Health Services Research Board that allocates funding for research into the provision of health care. In the past there was a tendency to believe that the only research worth funding was a randomized controlled trial, but a wider view of appropriate methods is now being taken. The MRC runs a number of grant application schemes running from 'small' grants of a few tens of thousands of pounds up to large 'programme' grants that might run to hundreds of thousands of pounds.
4. The BMA gives some research grants.
5. Various charities can be approached. For example, well-known for their contribution to medical research are the Nuffield Hospitals Provincial Trust and the Wellcome Foundation. There are also the more illness-specific charities such as the British Diabetic Association and the cancer charities. There are lots of others, sometimes only small, but then often overlooked. Your local postgraduate library should have one of the directories of charities which fund research.
6. The Department of Health funds research in health service delivery.

These various funds require different formats for the application, though most follow the usual protocol format outlined above. The precise requirements can be obtained by enquiring from the funding body itself. Your application will be sent out for referees' comments (just like a paper submitted to a journal) and on the basis of these comments the fund will make its decision. Remember that this process takes time and depends very much on the speed of the referees and how frequently the fund meets to allocate grants. Bear in mind that in many cases an informal approach to the fund can help your progress; sometimes you will be advised of subjects or areas which the fund is currently interested in funding, or you might learn of a useful way of couching your application. Sometimes fund-giving bodies will negotiate with applicants, so this is worth trying.

SUMMARY

This chapter has described how to prepare a research protocol which can act as your research map or as the basis for an application for funding.

SUGGESTED TASK

Why not start doing some research?

ANSWER TO EXERCISE

EXERCISE 11.1: REFERRAL RATE PROTOCOL

Aim: To establish my referral rate to hospital outpatients over a typical month in the practice.

Method: A referral rate requires a numerator and a denominator. The numerator will be all those patients referred to hospital outpatients during September. This will exclude patients simply sent to use hospital laboratories or those sent to A and E. The denominator will be all those patients who consult with me during surgeries and home visits.

A daily schedule will be prepared on which will be noted the age and sex of all patients consulting together with whether or not they were referred to hospital outpatients.

The numbers of patients consulting and the number referred will be calculated from the 30 schedules collected during September. Dividing the latter by the former and multiplying by 100 will give my referral rate per 100 patients consulting.

12 Doing audit

The past few years has seen greater and greater attention being concentrated on medical audit in general practice. In many ways the techniques required for audit are very similar to those used in research. This final chapter therefore addresses the ways in which knowledge of research methods can be used to further audit in primary health care.

THE POLITICS OF AUDIT

Research into health care over the last decade or so has revealed a remarkable feature of clinical activity in both primary health care and hospital, namely the large variation between individual clinicians even when caring for the same or similar sorts of patients. The considerable variability in prescribing and referral patterns in general practice is but one facet of this phenomenon. This variability is a cause of concern on two accounts. First, it is argued, the treatment any patient receives is determined by the chance of who happens to be providing it: surely this cannot mean that all patients are getting the most appropriate treatments. Second, this variability has considerable financial implications. At a time when health service resources seem under such pressure, the wide variations in clinical practice do suggest that some clinicians at least are being wasteful.

There are a number of responses to this problem. One, of course, is to pursue further research into good practice. Given that most therapies in medicine have not been properly evaluated there is a lot of work to do in this area—and having reached the last chapter of this book you may be able to contribute! However, even when one therapy is shown to be better than another, the evidence is that many clinicians continue to use the relatively ineffective one. The problem here is doctors' behaviour and this is where audit comes in.

Doctors learn at medical school, in postgraduate training, and throughout their professional lives. On the basis of this knowledge they practice medicine to the best of their ability. This freedom to apply their knowledge in the best interests of their patients is known as 'clinical autonomy'. In essence, clinical autonomy stresses the individuality of the doctor—in learning new knowledge, in applying that knowledge, in reviewing patients' welfare, and in revising knowledge and practice in the light of these outcomes. However, as this individuality has led to such variation in clinical practice, those outside the profession are taking an increasing interest in clinical freedom.

Telling doctors what they should do is one strategy, but it means the loss of those features of clinical freedom that can benefit the individual patient. The compromise is medical audit in which doctors themselves, without interference, share their knowledge and agree common standards of care. In this way they can preserve some autonomy yet at the same time reduce variability and improve care.

Certainly, on becoming a principal in general practice there is a need to rely on one's own professional integrity as an individual and independent GP to monitor performance. For most of the time this is, no doubt, an effective procedure but without some form of formal monitoring it is easy to believe that standards are being achieved when in fact they are not. It might be agreed that the reduction of high blood pressures in middle age will lower the incidence of strokes. But have all patients over the age of 50 years had their blood pressure checked and recorded in the notes? It is easy to say 'yes' or 'probably', but only by checking a sample of notes can it be properly confirmed. Thus an important part of audit is reviewing performance against agreed standards. More and more often, the government is seeing the attainment of targets as a means of reimbursing GPs for some aspects of care. Targets are nothing more than centrally determined standards of care. Have 80 per cent of the women aged 20 to 65 had a cervical smear within the past 5 years? If you have reached this standard of care, we'll pay you some extra money!

And what if standards are not being met? Well, if the standards are reasonable ones the implication is that something has got to change. If the standards are those attached to extra payments, implication may turn into obsession! This is where continuing medical education and practice management/organization skills come to the fore.

In overview then, audit is about enabling the processes of medicine to be carried out in a more rigorous and effective manner. Why not think about what changes are necessary in a more rigorous manner? Why not go for change with predictable benefits?

THE AUDIT CYCLE

Audit is concerned with monitoring performance against established standards, and implementing appropriate change, as necessary, to meet those standards.

Audit is usually described in terms of a cycle or spiral:

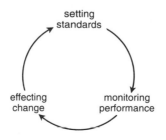

The cycle starts with the choice of a suitable area to scrutinize. It goes on to determine a standard that you feel should be achieved. Further around the circle, you have to measure what you are doing against your chosen standard. If you find that you are reaching that standard, then no problem, choose another topic and carry on. If, as is often the case, the standard is not being reached then it will be necessary to change that particular area so as to be able to reach the standard you have set yourself. The final stage will be to measure again at a later date to ensure that you are now, after the changes, reaching the standard.

There is nothing drastic, nothing revolutionary, and nothing that need be unduly threatening. There is indeed nothing that cannot be achieved by careful thought and choice of a topic and it is probable that this is precisely what you currently do 'in your head' in your professional work. Audit simply analyses the process more rigorously and makes it more explicit.

STANDARD SETTING

Choosing a topic

Having decided to audit some aspect of your practice where do you start? What should you look at first?

Chapter 1 described some approaches to selecting suitable questions for research. In a similar way, many of the same considerations, such as the question being sufficiently important and possible to answer, hold for audit topics. In addition there is another aspect that will need to be considered. Audit has a more practical side to it than pure research. An intrinsic part of the whole process is to introduce whatever changes are necessary to attain the agreed standards of care. If this is neither possible nor feasible then this would affect the choice of a particular problem.

Ask yourself: What exactly is my practice? What is wrong with my practice? General practice is a huge, dynamic organism, a complicated mixture of people, places, actions, and outcomes. The huge scope that it offers in the way of subject areas to audit can in itself be very daunting and inhibiting at the outset. There are, however, some processes that will direct you into selecting useful fields. To introduce order from the apparent disorder, the first task is to draw up a large list of possibilities and then to narrow the choice down using a list of criteria that will differentiate the possible from the fantastic, the useful from the theoretical.

Where do you get the long list from? Again, using a little thought and a little organization, the task becomes much easier. Breaking a large system into smaller more manageable parts can allow problem areas to be more readily focused upon. One way might be to divide general practice into three areas:

• clinical
• administrative
• business.

Any division is arbitrary, and there are probably many other ways of sub-dividing the work. The point of the exercise is allow one to narrow the task down to manageable size and then to look at each of these smaller areas in turn in order to develop the list.

Another approach would be to look at health care in terms of structure, process, and outcome. Structure consists of the framework of health care delivery—the buildings, the equipment, the personnel, the medical records. Process looks at what actually happens within the system and would include prescribing, investigation, and referral behaviour, and any part of the system where decisions are taken and actions implemented. Outcome is the measurable end-result of health care (from using some process within the structure). It is by far the most difficult area to look at and that is where audit and basic research so clearly overlap and inter-relate. Many of the actions undertaken in the name of health care have unknown outcomes in terms of prevention of illness or improvement in the level of patient autonomy.

Once the overall work of general practice has been in some way subdivided, the identification of suitable subjects within those areas can be further simplified by structuring and understanding the process of selection. The most useful areas to audit will be those in which a problem has been identified.

Practice problems

It is likely that the most fruitful source of topics will arise from within your own practice. These will be areas that have been recognized as being of concern to someone. How can you identify these 'buzz points'? One of the simplest ways would be to set up some form of 'death and disaster review' that will throw up problem areas. This model follows directly on from reviews of perinatal deaths that obstetricians and paediatricians have set up in many hospitals. You may decide that any complaint made by a patient will be considered through this process. All deaths from terminal cancer, or all deaths in under 60s, may again provide cases which, when considered, will produce ideas that could be suitable for audit and inclusion on the list.

Other topic areas may be identified from information that is now routinely supplied to GPs. A Level 3 analysis of PACT data, which can be requested from the Prescription Pricing Authority, might give some ideas about suitable prescribing areas. Prescribing targets will similarly provide possibilities.

Probably the richest source of ideas will come from discussion among members of the practice. The involvement of others is important even at this early stage: audit must be seen as a practice activity. It is not just 'your' little scheme, but something which is and will become a basic part of the practice infrastructure. It cannot be emphasized too often that it is vital that all members of staff are invited to be involved in all aspects of audit. As well as providing further examples, their involvement will greatly increase the likelihood that any data collection during the audit, and any necessary changes decided upon as a result of the exercise, will succeed. As stressed earlier, audit is about programmed change and anything that facilitates this change should be encouraged.

So how best to encourage suggestions from within the practice?

1. One way would be to organize 'brain storming' sessions with partners or other members of staff. Anything and everything can be put forward for consideration and discussion. It might usefully be combined with a meeting to discuss the whole question of what audit is all about.

2. Alternatively you might wish to follow up an exploratory session with perhaps a simple questionnaire to all members of staff asking for ideas. Whatever the method chosen, you will find that they will have views on problems within the system of which you are blissfully ignorant—habitual late starts to surgeries, perceived overwork, irate patients, and poor or confused communication between patients, staff and doctors.

3. Another simple method of identifying problems is to encourage everyone in the practice to write down anything that is considered to be a problem. This might be a clinical uncertainty in the consulting room—have all my hypertensives had their blood pressures taken and recorded within the last 6 months? It might be administrative—there were 6 people standing in the waiting room at 10 a.m. today. It might be business: how does my night visit income compare with others (am I claiming for all visits)? These lists can then be collected and combined, or act as a discussion point for a brain storming meeting.

National problems

From time to time—and probably increasingly more often as audit becomes a nationally identified high-profile area—problems in health care provision are identified by national or regional bodies. There has been a great deal of concern at the failure to reduce deaths from asthma over the past decade, despite the availability of better prophylactic treatments. Chest physicians have published reports suggesting that the management of this important clinical condition is less than adequate. Similar comments have been made about diabetics, multiple prescribing for the elderly, over-prescribing of antibiotics for URTIs, low immunization rates against influenza in at-risk groups, and so on. Barely a month goes by without an article appearing in the popular or medical press identifying some aspect of medical care in general practice that could be improved. Read the medical journals, national newspapers and weekly magazines to pick up these areas of concern and ask the question 'Does this criticism apply to me?'. For the time being, put the problem down on your list.

District problems

It could well be that problem areas will be identified by the local Medical Audit Advisory Group and that they will be circulating ideas to local GPs to consider. These problems may be national ones as above, or more local such as the length of waiting lists, the quality of referral letters, the adequacy of staff training. They may or may not be topics that you find interesting or wish to be involved in.

Working alone or within a small practice has its advantages in terms of independence and flexibility, but there can be a cost in terms of isolation and possible lack of rigour. Working as part of a district group will allow greater access to possible resources, including local expertise in audit, and the general support that may be required at the cost of reduced individual control. Problems shared by other practices will enable you to learn from their experiences and ideas. Take district-wide problems seriously and add them to the list.

Establishing standards

The most distinctive characteristic of audit is the monitoring of performance against some standard with a view to implementing change. Often what are put forward as audit exercises are little more than simple counting exercises. Although important in their own right in trying to describe general practice, they are not audit exercises as defined above. Sometimes, to move measurement towards audit, standards are assumed that have little basis in empirical studies of good practice. The assumption is made that in some way high prescribing is a 'bad thing' and sufficient variation in this direction from the local or national average for other GPs may result in a visit from the FHSA medical director. It is unlikely that a GP whose prescribing is of a similar aberrant nature, but in a 'low' direction, will receive commensurate attention. An implied standard that average means good and high means bad has been made, with little if any evidence to support it. Similar comments can be made in relation to investigation and referral rates. What does 'high' or 'low' mean in terms of the quality of patient care? How can one meaningfully decide a standard for these aspects of GP behaviour? The emphasis in the recent past has been on this type of blind process audit, whereas in years to come probably the most important aspect of audit will be the standard-setting exercise. Again there are risks that external bodies will intervene and attempt to 'impose' standards, but at the same time there are opportunities for GPs themselves to seize the initiative in this area and ensure that standards have relevance for everyday general practice and have the backing of local GPs.

There are a number of principles that should be followed when determining standards: the main ones are explicitness and viability.

Make standards explicit

In an important sense all doctors are engaged in audit every day in their professional work. This is because in their undergraduate and postgraduate education doctors learn professional values and standards of care on the basis of which they make clinical judgements. Thus, a patient with 'frequency' of micturition clearly fails to meet the 'norm' or standard which all doctors have been taught is part of a healthy life. The task of the practitioner is therefore to understand the reason for this and try and treat any underlying cause.

The problem with using this model of audit for reviewing performance is that the standards against which care is compared are implicit. This means that it is open to even the best-intentioned GP to create an illusion of good practice. Without laying out clearly what the standards of care aimed for actually are, it becomes all too easy to fudge the criteria when reviewing performance. A creative GP can always think of reasons why the standard should be different at the end of the review than before it. In effect, implicit standards do not provide a rigorous enough basis for a GP to carry out a proper self-evaluation to establish whether or not specific standards of care are being met.

The first rule of standard-setting is therefore that standards must be committed to paper to guard against self-deception. This is not an easy process but ensures that any standards so described are explicit and open to criticism and debate.

Choose viable topics

For many clinical problems, standards can be somewhat vague. For example, the ideal standard of outcome for a patient with backache is that they are cured of their problem, but in practice this can prove difficult; if a GP fails to meet this ideal standard this does not necessarily reflect on the quality of their care, but more on the limitations of available knowledge and treatments. Thus for many medical procedures the optimal outcome that can reasonably be expected is unknown, and therefore it is difficult to establish a precise standard against which to compare. This can mean that GPs are working to inappropriate standards. A GP may be satisfied with his or her management of backaches but might be applying a success criterion that is too low or unambitious. Equally, GPs may be applying standards that are unsupported by scientific evidence. For example, there is evidence that antibiotics are unnecessary for the treatment of much acute otitis media in children. However, many GPs still continue to prescribe in the mistaken belief that the standard to which they aspire is one of providing antibacterial drugs when an ear infection is identified.

It is easier to create standards for an area of clinical management for which 'hard evidence' on treatment exists. However, very often it is precisely those areas of medicine in which there is poor support or consensus for which standards are most helpful. Choice of topic therefore lies between stating the obvious and finding a way through the impossible.

Types of standard

The world of standards has much confusing jargon. Standards are often referred to as *protocols*. It has been suggested that it is useful to think in terms of options, guidelines, and standards, each offering less choice for the practitioner. Thus, *options*, which describe the range of acceptable treatments, may be appropriate for conditions which need flexibility in their management; *guidelines* describe how GPs should behave in most instances; and finally *standards* have a ring of absoluteness about them. However, standards themselves can contain flexibility in as much as they are often expressed as the percentage of an underlying *criterion*. Thus a criterion might be that all patients with diabetes should have their feet inspected once a year, but accepting that GPs work in the real world, the standard might be that 90 per cent of patients with diabetes should have their feet inspected once a year.

An important feature of standards is that they are usually written down, so that when performance is reviewed there can be no mistake about the criteria against which they are to be compared. There are different forms of standards or protocols available. Some may take the form of an algorithm which sets out the precise steps to be followed at each stage of a process. Others, more like guidelines or options, might provide recommendations or rules which should be followed. The latter should be flexible, coherent, and revisable. Attention should be paid to the layout of the protocol and to its length. In the final analysis it is against the chosen standard that performance will be compared and therefore it should be such that compliance can be measured.

Standards can be divided into three types, depending on how they were created.

Self-generated standards

GPs are still independent individuals and therefore they may wish to carry out self-audit and generate their own standards of care. In effect this is a further step up from the implicit standards which govern much of professional practice. The major difference is that here the standards of care must be written down. This enables individual GPs to see in a more objective way the sorts of norms which they are setting for themselves and the standard of care they are aiming to provide.

Of course, the opportunity for self-deception is still present in that if subsequently performance is found not to meet the standards, it requires a very determined and disciplined approach to offer appropriate self-criticism and institute corrective action. In addition, there is a likelihood that such individually devised standards may be inappropriate or, at least, poorly devised and set out. This possibility can be minimized to some degree by obtaining the views of others on these self-derived standards. Thus a GP who describes the standards of care which he or she will provide for antenatal patients would be wise to show the initial draft to other GP colleagues to obtain their views. In practice this is a most important step because it is only with the critical comments of others that the clarity of standards can be properly established.

Group-derived standards

Involving other GPs in commenting on a set of standards leads naturally to the much more common technique of preparing standards as a group.

Many of the clinical protocols or guidelines which have been prepared for use in general practice have arisen through GPs working in such groups, which may comprise partners, young principals' group, trainers' workshops, or may even extend to a district-wide or area-wide involvement. Group-derived standards have the advantage that they have been subjected to critical appraisal by a number of different clinicians. They will more likely reflect commonly agreed 'good practice' than the idiosyncratic views of one GP. It is also likely, if they are to be understood by all GP members of the group, that they will be clear and explicit.

Setting standards as a group can itself be a rewarding task. The very process of arguing through what the standards should be—drawing upon personal experience and scientific evidence—is an educational exercise and in itself may produce changes in clinical behaviour.

The main problem with creating group standards lies in this very interchange between different GPs of differing views. Achieving consensus can be difficult and 'compromise' standards are not necessarily the best. Techniques for resolving this conflict are discussed below.

Standards created by others

One of the functions of professional organizations is to help maintain good standards of care across their specialty. This has led Royal Colleges and other professional bodies to enter the field of standard-setting. The process by which such standards are created is through expert committees, who will draw upon the evidence, discuss, and pronounce on the best available care. Again, such committees themselves can be divided, especially over controversial areas of medicine, and one approach has been to develop 'consensus conferences' when a panel, after hearing the evidence, are required to reach a consensus statement on what is the best quality of care.

Standards established by groups of experts have an important part to play in the audit process. Their advantage is that they are usually based on the most up-to-date knowledge and reflect 'state of the art' judgements. However, experts can be far removed from the coal-face of general practice and it is not impossible for such standards to be unrealistic or inappropriate for the day-to-day routines of the average GP. Moreover, the major disadvantage of expert-derived standards is that individual GPs rarely feel any sense of ownership or involvement with the standards. GPs are going to be less likely to review their performance and even less likely to institute change, on the basis of standards to which they feel no commitment or trust. The great strength of standards prepared by groups of GPs is that the participating doctors are more likely to feel a sense of involvement and commitment than if the standards, even nominally better, are handed down from others.

Obtaining consensus

Standards can be set by local GPs—a practice, a number of practices, or GPs from an area—getting together and agreeing a common approach to some area of work. In the main these gatherings involve participants discussing the issues in an attempt to reach consensus. Sometimes the agreement comes easily, sometimes there are serious differences; sometimes everyone is involved, sometimes some views are ignored or excluded. Much depends on the participants and the dynamics of the meeting. However, this process can equally be approached as a research problem.

Question

What is the research question?

- How can consensus be best achieved?
- What is the best level of agreement that can be achieved with this group of GPs?
- What set of standards is likely to achieve the widest support?

The exact question will depend on the size and scope of the standard-setting exercise. For a small practice-based problem it may be rather limited; but for a district-wide process, perhaps involving a hundred GPs, then it certainly merits being addressed with the rigours of a research project.

Method

There are a number of methods that can be used to help develop a consensus.

1. The principles of qualitative method in preliminary discussions with colleagues to identify recurrent themes—perhaps issues on which there is agreement and those on which there is dissent.
2. 'Snowballing' involves GPs working in pairs to discuss the draft protocol and any amendments which they feel they themselves would require. These pairs then contribute their thoughts to a smaller group of GPs which again tries to reach some degree of agreement. These separate groups then come together either as a plenary or through their representatives to establish what consensus has emerged.
3. A nominal group approach, which is a sort of structured group meeting that allows everyone to contribute and feel some 'ownership' of the result (see Fig. 12.1).
4. A questionnaire to colleagues based on a draft list of standards inviting their comments on those they would be willing to support and those about which they have doubts.
5. The Delphi technique, in which GPs in a defined group are sent the draft protocol by post with an invitation to evaluate it. The responses are then amalgamated to produce a revised draft which is likely to be more acceptable to GP members of the group. This again is returned to all GPs for their further comments. This process continues until an agreed protocol emerges (see Fig. 12.2).

No doubt there are many other ways of creatively obtaining consensus from your colleagues, especially in getting views or responses to views by questionnaire. Many of the topics discussed in previous chapters, such as questionnaire design and data analysis, may be found useful in this process.

Conclusion

Establishing standards is an important procedure in the process of carrying out audit. It is not simply a brief preliminary in this process but requires considerable

Invite all members of a group to write down, say, five things that they consider to be the most important features of some problem, perhaps the care of asthmatics. Each in turn is invited to describe their first priority which is then written on a flip chart. The second most important item is then taken from each member of the group and written down. This happens until all the items are aired.

Each item from the overall list is discussed. This is followed by everyone scoring the group items—perhaps in order of priority, or level of agreement—using a convenient scoring system (say, everyone has five 'votes' to distribute). The result is a list of items derived and prioritized by all members of the group.

Although the technique might seem rather elaborate, it is easy to use in practice. It ensures that everyone contributes their own ideas, that all ideas are discussed, and that everyone has a say in the final result. For obtaining a consensus on some controversial issue the technique has much to commend it.

Fig. 12.1 Nominal groups.

Post a draft set of standards to a group of GPs (perhaps all the GPs in a health district). The respondents are invited to express their views in some way. On returning the questionnaires, the responses are aggregated and the average (and perhaps range of values for all GPs) is sent back to all respondents in a second mailing. Again all GPs are invited to provide their views, but this time in the context of seeing the views of their colleagues. What tends to happen is that views now shift towards greater agreement as outliers readjust their assessments. This process— a sort of iterative consensus conference—can go on for several rounds but there are diminishing returns, and respondents can get weary. Nevertheless, the Delphi technique is a useful way of involving everyone in decision-making without requiring them all to meet together.

Fig. 12.2 Delphi technique.

thought and effort to be carried out satisfactorily. If it is a standard which is devised by a group of GPs then the process of arriving at this standard will itself be an important educational activity which may have a considerable impact on clinical practice whether or not performance is reviewed in future against the standard.

The standards in the form of guidelines or protocols prepared by a group of GPs are only provisional. Medical knowledge changes rapidly, and it is likely that the standard will need regular revising. It is important to recognize this by placing the date of completion in a prominent position on the protocol. This will remind GPs using it of its provenance and of the need to revise it in years to come.

MONITORING PERFORMANCE

The central part of any audit exercise is the collection of data. Without this, you will be unable to compare against the standards you have set yourself. Details of many aspects of data definition, collection, and analysis have been described in earlier chapters. Here it is only necessary to highlight those points in respect of an audit exercise that merit repetition.

Temporal aspects

The way that the data are collected has important implications for interpretation and usefulness. It is clear that one can collect information about events that have occurred in the past—a retrospective analysis, or plan to collect them as they happen in the future—prospective analysis.

Retrospective data collection

Into this category fall the 'death and disaster' type of case review discussed earlier. Similarly an audit of diabetic care as recorded in the notes is an analysis of your behaviour in the past against standards you have just decided upon. Obviously this retrospective assessment can cause problems, for example if the standard of record keeping in the notes has been poor, but it is often easier to organize.

Prospective data collection

Collecting data 'on the run' can ensure that all the necessary pieces of data can be accumulated but does suffer the disadvantage that the audit exercise itself might have an effect that could influence opinions and behaviour and give a less than true picture.

Samples

One question that must be addressed before starting to collect data is that of the number of cases. In an ideal world one would collect data from all possible cases, that is from the whole of what is described as the target population. However, there are limits to time, patience, and resources. Therefore it is likely that there will be a limit to the number of cases that you will want, or indeed will be able, to collect. If the audit involves a fairly discrete, easily identifiable group, such as all patients diagnosed as having diabetes, then it may be possible to look at the whole group. All that will remain will be to design a method of identifying them—easy if you have a reasonably accurate computer system or disease register, but also possible through the repeat prescription system if you have not.

You may, on the other hand, have decided to audit your prescriptions for legibility, presence of clear instructions, and quantity to be dispensed. You could do this by looking at all the prescriptions you have ever written—clearly a ludicrous suggestion, but one that would give you the most perfect result. The pragmatic compromise is to look at a sample of your prescriptions, such as those written within the past month, on the assumption that the past month is a reasonable snapshot of your behaviour and that it was fairly typical in terms of what you did in any other month in the past. Chapters 2 and 8 discussed ways of ensuring that the number collected does in fact give a fair representation of your overall behaviour, but at the end of the day one has to make a pragmatic judgement that enough is enough. Clearly analysing one or two prescriptions is unlikely to give a fair impression, one or two hundred much more likely to. The greater the number, the smaller the likely error. However, in audit the goal is not statistical significance but clinical implication: some result might be 'significant' at the $p < 0.001$ level but be unimportant in everyday practice. For audit, the restraints of time and effort will be greater determinants of number than will any statistical model.

Record cards or schedules

Whatever way you decide to collect and organize your data, thought must be given as to how you are going to record the information so as to able to analyse it and compare with your standards. The best way of doing this is to design a schedule. What do these look like?

Dr Andy Chronical has decided to audit the clinical records of his adult asthmatics. He decides that among an appropriate set of standards are:

- all records should contain a peak flow recording within the past 6 months
- all records should contain present smoking history
- all records should contain a family history, etc.

His recording schedule should ideally be a single sheet of paper for each case. It should contain a title. The first entry would probably be the patient's name and possibly a code number. He might want the date on which he collects the data and places to record the data extracted from the notes. It would look something like this:

Asthma Audit Schedule

Name: Number: Date:

	Yes	No
Peak flow in last 6 months		
Smoking history recorded		
Family history asthma recorded		
Inhaler technique checked in 6 months		

The advantage of such a schedule is that nothing is forgotten and the data are not spread out over bits and pieces of paper. Time spent in designing a clear schedule will more than repay itself in the ease with which the information can be interpreted later.

Types of data collection

Case analysis

One of the easiest auditing exercises to set up is one which involves an analysis of case notes. Designing a concise schedule will make the task easy, but whether or not the information is recorded will cause the most frustration.

Questionnaires

Many of the audit exercises that involve asking opinions of second or third parties will involve the use of questionnaires. The design of these has been described in Chapter 4. The difficulty is trying to ensure that the questionnaire will achieve what you intend both in respect of the data it represents and also whether or not your target group will complete and return it. A 'good' questionnaire does not happen by chance and some of the more obvious pitfalls can be avoided as outlined earlier.

The pilot study

As with any other kind of research project one needs to be certain that the chosen method works before embarking on any data-collecting exercise. For that reason a pilot study or trial run may well save a great deal of time, effort, enthusiasm, and cooperation. There is no point in handing out 50 questionnaires to your patients if the questions are difficult to answer or so many that no one returns the form. Similarly, asking receptionists to record telephone calls received might be impossible during the middle of a busy morning surgery.

EFFECTING CHANGE

Change: to alter, convert, transform, modify, mutilate.

Changing behaviour is not an easy task. Doctors tend by nature to be conservative in their approach to their patients, their profession, and life in general. Changing physician behaviour is recognized as being extremely difficult.

Yet audit is all about change. It is about comparing present behaviour against standards and being willing to change that behaviour in order to bring yourself or your practice up towards those standards. It is the central purpose of the whole process. Without change, audit is a meaningless process of data collection.

Approaching change

There are several approaches that can be taken to get colleagues and staff to change.

Education

Attempts can be made to educate colleagues and staff into 'better' ways. This is the basis of all postgraduate educational events that aim to bring you up-to-date and then hopefully alter the way you do things in light of the new knowledge you have learned.

Feedback

Another way of trying to change the behaviour of doctors is through feedback mechanisms. The PACT exercise relies on this method by showing doctors their prescribing behaviour and allowing them to see how they compare with local and national peers. Consultant letters in response to referrals can be another avenue where comment and information about one aspect of your patient management may make you think about your approach to patients with similar problems in the future.

Financial reward

GPs can be bribed into changing behaviour. Establishing payments for attendance at postgraduate education events has led to a huge increase in the number of doctors going to lectures. Item of service payments serve the same purpose.

Financial penalties

GPs can be financially penalized into changing behaviour. The differential night visit fee attempts to dissuade GPs from opting to form large groups or using commercial deputizing cover to provide out-of-hours cover.

Participation

Another way of changing behaviour is to involve the target doctors in the change process. The argument is that you are more likely to be willing to change if you yourself have been one of the prime movers in deciding upon the change and have been fully involved in determining the reason and necessity for the change.

Administrative changes

Finally, change can be forced upon doctors by administrative changes. GPs can be required to carry out certain activities as part of the terms and conditions of service within the NHS.

Resistance to change

Yet resistance to change is often a stronger force than any of these approaches. As a profession, medicine likes to think that education and feedback should be the most likely and acceptable way of changing, but unfortunately there is evidence that these factors alone have little effect. It is administrative changes from outside, and also within, the profession that seem most likely to cause change. The spiralling cost of health care, the acknowledgment of the wide variation in behaviour such as prescribing and referral, and pressure to provide only reasonable and necessary treatments, underpin the whole encouragement of the audit process by the government. Its chances of success, and the degree of control the profession retains over it, will depend very much on their approach to it.

Achieving change

So how can change be accommodated and how can others be encouraged to change?

Be involved

The most basic requirement is for all those likely to be affected by changes to be involved in the audit process. If an audit of the telephone system has revealed long delays in answering and abruptness in manner as two areas for change, then telling the receptionists to answer the phone more quickly and to be more pleasant is highly unlikely to achieve a permanent improvement in these areas. If you find that only 10 per cent of hypertensive patients have had their fundi looked at in the past year, then requesting all partners to make sure that this is carried out and recorded at least annually is unlikely to improve the situation greatly.

If your receptionists, in the first instance, and partners, in the second, have been committed to the idea of the audit from the start through being made to feel part of all decisions and discussions, then they will have been involved in deciding what changes are necessary and therefore will be more likely to carry these through. They will have 'ownership' of the whole audit and so will accept the changes as being a necessary and integral part of it.

Choose a meaningful topic

In this context, meaningful means 'meaningful for those likely to be affected by changes'. The topic must be seen to be significant enough to justify any changes. The benefits must clearly outweigh the hassle for those involved. It is extremely important, as emphasized earlier, that the choice of topic is made with the full agreement of any practice staff likely to be involved. It is fundamental to the whole operation that the process leads to change, and it must be in the light of the level of agreement that final choices are made from the shortlist

Set suitable standards

Closely connected with the choice of topic is the setting of realizable standards. The standards must be appropriate for you and your practice. Everyone starts off from different baselines. Although there may be some 'gold standard' that can be aspired to, to achieve change the jumps forward must be sensible and achievable. Failing to reach targets can be very dispiriting; the converse is equally true. Whilst one might want 100 per cent of patients seen within 10 minutes of their appointment times, this is clearly incompatible with an efficient use of doctor consulting time. However, if your audit shows that only 20 per cent of patients are seen within this time period, it is possible that a standard of 50 per cent could be reached with minor changes and 75 per cent with some thought.

If, in the discussion of standards in relation to the management of hypertensive patients, one or more of your partners refuses to acknowledge the importance or necessity of yearly fundoscopy, then negotiate to persuade, accommodate to proceed, or recognize a fundamental problem and move to another area on which agreement can be reached on standards. Similarly, discussions right at the start with reception staff about the telephone system, their involvement in setting the standards for promptness of reply, helpful manner, and so on, will then make decisions about the necessary changes much easier. Indeed the general approach to necessary changes should be implicit in the standard-setting exercise and the choice of audit topic. Setting a standard which change would be unable to attain means that the standard is inappropriate. The whole audit process can be become a meaningless extra task if this part of the exercise is badly handled. Worse still, it might alienate partners and staff against the whole idea and make future exercises almost impossible to initiate.

Set an appropriate time scale for change

There is a fine balance between trying to do too much too soon and being so careful in introducing changes that initiative and enthusiasm are given time to leak away. The deciding factor will be the scale and type of the changes required. Again, the main requisite is discussion and involvement of those affected. Implicit in the audit process is the requirement to measure again after instituting changes. It is important to give sufficient time for the changes to be introduced and for the changes to have any effect.

Changing the content of referral letters to reach higher standards of legibility and information can be introduced over a relatively short time period—it is mainly a change in attitude that is required and this, if the points above have been followed, should have been achieved by this stage. A further audit after 3 months might be suitable.

Changing a whole appointment system to make it more flexible, sensitive to sudden surges of demand, and so on, is a much more complicated issue. There may be several different proposals put forward to try and these may be found to be impracticable. It is often possible to experiment initially with just one partner, or on one day a week.

Involve, discuss, and be sensitive to the effect the changes may be having.

Reward success

As described above, one way of introducing change is through financial rewards. This applies at all levels of staff and need not be grandiose. A one-off bonus might be the carrot for staff, if reaching a standard results in significant financial gain for the practice. Reaching a desired standard in patient satisfaction might warrant cracking open a couple of bottles of Bulgarian Chardonnay.

No successful audit should go by without some token of recognition.

SUMMARY

Audit is not the same as research, but the techniques of the latter can often be used to illuminate the former. Most of the issues described in the earlier chapters will be found to be of value in audit.

Audit is all about change: change for the better in a purposeful manner. It need not be a negative statutory requirement. It can be an extremely powerful weapon from which all can benefit. Probably the most difficult part of all will be introducing any changes that have been shown to be needed. A little thought, moderate tact, universal involvement, and open and continuing discussion should greatly increase the likelihood of success.

AUDIT TASKS

1. With your partners, practice and district nurses, and other relevant team members, discuss the management of the last two cases with terminal cancer in the practice. Identify the good points of the management and make a list of five areas where problems were experienced.

2. Call a meeting of practice staff and spend one hour brainstorming problems in the organization of the practice. Make a list of these areas.

3. Contact the Chairman of your local MAAG (get the number from the FHSA). Ask him or her for details of any local audits that are being proposed.

4. Draw up a list of five clinical, five administrative, and five business areas that might be suitable for audit.

5. With your district nurse identify a set of standards for the degree of involvement you have in the management of patients on your list she is presently treating. Design a schedule you could use for this audit.

6. Design a schedule for two of the audit projects you have selected with your team. Try them out in a small pilot study. Discuss the results with the team.

Index